Christ Walk

Christ Walk

A
40-Day
Spiritual
Fitness
Program

ANNA FITCH COURIE

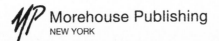

Morehouse Publishing
NEW YORK

For Emmanuel Church, Hampton, Virginia

Morehouse Publishing, 4785 Linglestown Road, Suite 101, Harrisburg, PA 17112
Morehouse Publishing, 19 East 34th Street, New York, NY 10016
Morehouse Publishing is an imprint of Church Publishing Incorporated.
www.churchpublishing.org

Cover design by Laurie Klein Westhafer
Interior design and typesetting by Beth Oberholtzer

Library of Congress Cataloging-in-Publication Data

Fitch Courie, Anna.
    Christ walk : a 40-day spiritual fitness program / Anna Fitch Courie.
      pages   cm
    Includes bibliographical references.
      ISBN 978-0-8192-3169-7 (pbk.)—ISBN 978-0-8192-3170-3 (ebook) 1. Health—Religious aspect—Christianity. 2. Walking—Religious aspects—Christianity. 3. Spiritual life--Christianity. I. Title.
BT732.F58 2014
248.4'6—dc22

                                                          2014025395

Printed in the United States of America

Contents

Part Three: Judgment

Part Four: Repentance

Part Five: Redemption

Appendices

Acknowledgments

The idea for Christ Walk began as a forty-day spiritual journey designed for Lent. God planted this seed in my head when I was not sure what I wanted to do with my life. Our church, Emmanuel Episcopal Church in Hampton, Virginia, gave me the opportunity and a church family in which to explore and test this theory for mind, body, and spiritual health through walking. For that, I thank them from the bottom of my heart. I would like to especially thank Father Derek Pringle. When I first approached Father Pringle with the idea of Christ Walk, I was brand new to Emmanuel Church and he was somewhat skeptical of how the program would be received. I am eternally grateful that he took a leap of faith and allowed me to offer Christ Walk. Thank you for your trust and faith! To the members of the first Christ Walk group: Karen, Boyd, Adrian, Chuck, Linda, Jack and Jan, Mary, Andy, Melanie, Becky, Jackie, Joy, Judy, Laura, Ginny, and Jane—thank you so much for asking me to write this book. I would also like to thank my work colleagues, as they taught me everything I know about health promotion. To my editor, Sharon, thank you. I'm so glad you picked Christ Walk for your project! To my informal editors, Jason and Treb—thank you. To my family and friends, especially Treb; my children Patton and Merryn, all my thanks and love for your encouragement and the TIME to make this happen. For Caroline who believes in this journey, thank you. For Carrie and Richard who said, "Yes, this will be published!" (and then recommended me to Church Publishing), thank you! Finally, all my thanks to God for giving me the spiritual guidance and tools to show others that health of the body is as much a gift of God as health of the spirit and mind.

Introduction

"Take a step of faith in Christ." —Father Derek Pringle, Emmanuel Episcopal Church

I am an average person. I am average weight, average height, average looks, average intelligence, average Christian, average person. I like to think I am normal, with normal issues as the average person, with the average struggles and the average thoughts, beliefs, doubts, concerns, wants, and needs. I believe that the average person finds it hard to find time for prayers, healthy eating, exercise, time with family, demands of job, and everything else that we "should" be doing. I believe that Christ-centered living can get us there. A Christ-centered life provides us with forgiveness when we slip up, or when we need extra help, or when we need a friend on the walk of life. Christ helps us transcend the average and ordinary, to reach the extraordinary. Since Christ lives in all of us, average is a misleading description. I believe that all of us have opportunities to improve our health and transform ourselves through Christ to the amazing and extraordinary. Christ Walk is a program towards a healthy, Christ-centered life. We use the grace of God and the strength of Jesus to improve our health: mind, body, and spirit.

Christ Walk began in 2006 at Emmanuel Episcopal Church in Hampton, Virginia. I remember walking into the priest's office just as bold as you please and telling him that I was going to run a walking program during the six weeks of Lent for the parishioners. Father Derek was either bowled over or incredibly trusting as he gave me the go-ahead to implement my program. That began an odyssey of implementing Christ Walk for multiple churches. I will always be incredibly thankful to Emmanuel for the gift of testing the Christ Walk Program with me. I pray that they received as much out of Christ Walk as I received in sharing it.

A registered nurse by training, I am married to an Army officer; my professional life has taken twists and turns depending upon where my husband has been stationed. While stationed in Germany I was unable to find a job as a nurse so ended up landing a position as a health promotion coordinator for the 1ˢᵗ Infantry Division and Würzburg Medical Command. It was a life-changing and career-changing experience for me as I found that helping people become healthier was the calling in life that I always wanted. When we moved back to the States following our tour in Germany, I was seven months pregnant and had given up my dream job. I was not sure what I was going to do, but felt this strong calling to develop a walking program for my church. I had done something similar with the 1ˢᵗ Infantry Division by developing the "Walk to Iraq and Back" program for deployed spouses. The "Walk to Iraq and Back" program was a yearlong walking initiative designed for spouses of soldiers deployed to Iraq to walk the miles to Iraq and back over the course of deployment. From that experience, I knew the routes in the Bible would make for an incredible fitness experience. Thus "Christ Walk" grew out of my experience with health promotion programming, but centered on walking with Christ every day. I believe we need to exercise in mind, body, and spirit in order to make a body strong and whole.

The Bible has a great deal of inspiration for living healthy in mind, body, and spirit. As a result, you will find quotations from the Bible at the beginning of every chapter of this book. While I generally do not like "cherry picking" biblical verses outside of the context of the story, I have found that these phrases have been guideposts to ensure that Christ Walk stays centered on God. You may have other verses that call you to a healthy life, but I hope and pray that these verses will lift you up on your own Christ Walk journey.

I am an Episcopalian, although I feel quite comfortable in a variety of churches and have heard God's Word in many denominations outside of my own. Christ Walk is not intended to be just for Episcopalians; however, there will be references to the church year and church traditions that will be familiar to those from a liturgical tradition. Christ Walk was originally designed for the forty days of Lent, a time when many take on a spiritual discipline. However, Christ Walk can be used in any 40-day period.

Forty days is a powerful period of time in the Bible, and Lent is often used as a time of prayer, fasting, denial, and personal goals as we prepare ourselves for the forgiveness God gives us in Jesus' resurrection. Forty days can be transformational. While you can do Christ Walk at any forty-day period during the year, I find it an especially powerful tool during Lent. My Christ Walk challenge reminds me to always be cognizant of walking with Christ every day of my life.

I have also designed this book to be written in for you to track the progress on your journey and express your thoughts about your mind, body, and spirit. Research shows that people who journal about their health and their progress towards their goals are more likely to stick to their plans. People who track their goals are more likely to be successful in their endeavors. Christ Walk is not just for reading. Christ Walk is for living.

In each chapter (day) you will find a space to record your physical accomplishments with the exercise you have completed, the thoughts that you have discovered, and the spiritual insights you have experienced as a part of your Christ Walk journey. Christ Walk is designed to be shared, recorded, used, and reused as every day of walking with Christ is a new experience and new revelation into a healthier life.

I am passionate about God's presence in all of our lives, including my own. I was born in 1975 in Asheville, North Carolina, the daughter of an Episcopal priest who served as a Navy chaplain. I have a double-bogey against me: a preacher's kid (PK) and a Navy brat! But I think I turned out all right. My parents brought my brother and me up in the church. I have always believed in God, but my belief was more of the status quo rather than an active experience of my daily life.

During my teens, there were two major events that resulted in a powerful connection with God and the birth of my spirituality as I know it today. My father began suffering from mental illness, and he deteriorated over the next ten to fifteen years until he ended up having a stroke at the age of fifty-six. During that same period, I unexpectedly lost my hearing to an autoimmune disease. The doctors were not sure what was causing my hearing loss and associated symptoms, putting me on many experimental therapies in order to stem the hearing loss. Despite these efforts, I lost the remainder of my hearing at the age of fifteen and went through a six-month period completely deaf. I remember very vividly being in church one Sunday as we all stood to say the Nicene Creed. I could not hear anything. I sat down suddenly, extremely angry, frustrated, sad, and fed up that I could not hear the words of the service. I remember thinking, "Why bother?" and "What's the point if I cannot hear and participate?" Then I remember very clearly the voice of the Lord saying, "It does not matter, you don't have to *hear* to *experience*." And a light went on for me. I do not have to hear, I do not have to do this by rote, but I do have to experience God's love and share God's love with all that I am, however I am. We are all different, with our own losses and own pains, and we can ALWAYS experience God's love and share God's love with others, because he is the living God here on earth. What matters is how we love and how we use our bodies and lives towards God's love.

That is my spiritual strength. God gave me a message that has endured through various ups and downs and tragedies; we all have a place in doing

God's work in the world no matter how we are built or with what faulty equipment we are endowed. I know without a doubt that God is here amongst us and shares in our everyday lives. When I have the most internal conflict over my life, it is invariably because I am paying too much attention to the self, rather than what God is telling me. We are not put on this earth to focus on the SELF, rather what the self can do for *God*.

My mental strength is my ability to reason, to always search for knowledge and growth. I probably find this my easiest place of growth because I love to learn and read. However, for you it may be your challenge, and during Christ Walk you may set a learning goal as a part of your journey. Your ability to learn never ends. In fact, I think sometimes our ability to learn improves as we age when we put our minds to it.

I have never felt strong physically. My body always feels like it is against me. I am not a very athletic person, nor a very competitive person. I have asthma and allergies, gastrointestinal problems, hearing loss, and one leg that is a bit shorter than the other. I often feel that when I set a physical goal (I have now run three half marathons and a ten-miler, none of which seemed easy) that something invariably happens with my body to keep me from being successful (or what I have defined as successful in my own mind). One of the great lessons in life that I continue to learn is that success in my mind may not be the same as success in God's mind. I have learned that my physical strength is to never give up. Each day is an opportunity for me to strengthen my body in some way.

With Christ Walk, my goal for you is to set mind, body, and spirit goals that will help you focus on God. Take care of the temple (the body) that God has given us for the Christ spark in us all. We are all different. We are all different shapes and sizes and all different levels of health, wellness, and physical capability, but we all have a bit of Christ within us. Therefore we should take care of the temple that God has given us. A healthy body can do more for others and share the Christ love within us in whatever capacity we are called to serve.

Finally, these are my thoughts, feelings, beliefs and experiences. I will use a lot of "I" statements, since my experiences have shaped my theological beliefs on the topic of health and wellness. If these thoughts and feelings and beliefs do not resonate with your own experience, that is okay. All of our experiences collectively are shaping the Christian community's testament to God in the world. It is all good when it is done for the love of Christ. I hope that these meditations help you along on your journey. I hope you feel free to make it your own so that it works within your own set of thoughts, feelings, beliefs, and experiences. It is all good in the Spirit of God.

So, through strong minds, strong bodies, and strong spirits, we can walk with Christ all the days of our lives. Join me over the next forty days on your personal Christ Walk experience and see yourself transformed.

My physical goal for Christ Walk the next forty days is:

Dont Quit

My spiritual goal for Christ Walk the next forty days is:

Get closer to God, focus on Him and others instead of myself

My mental goal for Christ Walk the next forty days is:

Don't focus on other's judgement or opinions

PART ONE

Creation

March 1 An Introduction to Christ Walk

BIBLICAL BIG IDEA #1

Walk in love, as Christ loved us and gave himself up for us.
—Ephesians 5:2a

What is Christ Walk? Christ Walk is a spiritual fitness program. It is designed to improve your physical health, although anyone at any fitness or health level can participate in the program. I have a list of biblical routes (Appendix A) for you to choose a biblical journey to walk, run, bike, or pray (the distance of) during the next forty days. There is a chapter a day (Day 1, Day 2, etc.) to help lift you up spiritually as you make your journey.

In writing this book, I do not claim to be an expert on what is the best thing for you to do to have a spiritually and physically healthy life. I am not a theologian, although from my studies I would argue that anyone who studies and works towards a closer relationship with God could be considered a theologian. I do not claim to have all the answers. Much like any Christian, I have many questions that I constantly seek answers for, which to me is an act of faith. I am not an expert on health, although I have worked in the healthcare field for the last seventeen years with an emphasis on health programs and training. I do not claim that this book is the answer to all of the questions that you may have. It is not a diet, nor a guidebook, nor even a recommendation on how you should live.

This book is a personal reflection on my experiences, beliefs, and knowledge on having a spiritually and physically healthy life. After six years of running a Christ Walk program at several churches that was well received and provided an opportunity for the participants to grow spiritually and physically, I decided to share the program with others. The book in your hands is a manual/journal for you to have an interactive experience in the Christ Walk journey, much as the participants in my classes experienced! At the end of the forty days, this book should be as much your book as it is mine. Individuals as well as groups can use it. The appendices include options for group leaders and options for individuals to transform their Christ Walk experience from journey to journey. There is always another journey. Christ Walk should not end after one forty-day period. These forty days should transform you to pursue new journeys and new goals.

The Bible is filled with stories about journeys and food and eating and celebration. God did not intend for us to be at war with food, nor did he intend for us *not* to use our feet and our bodies in our daily lives. I am filled with awe that Christianity spread during a time when there were no cars, or trucks, or trains, or airplanes to get our prophets and disciples to the places where they wanted to spread the word. There is a reason God gave us feet! We have feet to walk, run, jump, and skip through our lives. Our feet are to be used to care for the temple God created within each of us.

When I have struggled with how to live my life, for the strength to get out and exercise when all I want to do is stay at home, or when I have been conflicted by the stresses in my life, I have always felt that God was there to help me and provide me with strength and guidance. I remember running my first half marathon. Around mile nine I began to fail and doubt. I began to pray that God would wrap my legs in strength and endurance. I felt the power of the Holy Spirit lift my legs and make them strong again. I truly believe God's strength helped me finish my race. The belief that I was not alone rejuvenated me. I believe that God walks with me in every step that I take. I believe that the Bible is filled with inspirational guidelines on living a healthy life. Through the next forty days, I would like to share that with you, as well as sharing a bit of my life and my journey through Christ Walk.

Each day, there will be a Bible verse related to a reflective piece on healthy living. Some of these days may be more body-focused and other days may be more spiritually or mentally focused. All of these days will help you on your journey to a healthier you! If you are physically unable to walk, I ask that you look at your life for ways that you can change it and improve it. We all have things that we can do to make our lives healthier. Perhaps your goal will be to study something new on your journey, or to pray with more discipline or to focus on changing your nutritional habits. If you cannot physically exercise, discuss with your health care provider some options that you are willing to do to improve your health. There is a place in this journey for everyone. We may need to be creative about how the journey is completed. I ask that you pray through those chapters that are not applicable to you and really focus on the ones that speak to your personal experience. I have tried to write to many different perspectives and needs. I am aware that this book will not work for everyone, but if you cannot make the journey on your own, consider how you can help others on their journey. Keep an open mind and again, consider, "What can I do to change?"

So how do we make a healthy body? We take care of it. We exercise it, we feed it, we nurture it, and we rest it. Research has documented on multiple occasions that walking is one of the most physically beneficial exercises, as well as one that people are most likely to stick to over time. Most of the journeys in the Bible were done by foot. Consequently, as you begin this journey with me, I am going to ask you to pick a walking goal (see Appendix A) to focus on during the next forty days. There are different walking goals depending on your fitness level. Some people have walked the *Via Dolorosa* (Jesus' journey through Jerusalem to his crucifixion, one of my favorite routes), others walked Jesus' birth and death (the distance between Bethlehem and Jerusalem), while others have walked Paul's missionary journeys. There is a complete list of suggested journeys and distances for you to set for your goal (Appendix A). Or you may choose to set your own goal! It is up to you. But as we physically walk through our Christ Walk journey, it will help to focus you on your spiritual goals as well.

Through Christ Walk, we have taken our daily journey as members of the Body of Christ, and translated that to actual physical walking goals that are pulled from routes that Jesus and the disciples took during varying missions. You can find a breakdown of each of these routes and their miles in the Appendices. Some of these distances are estimates. At the time I developed the routes, I was using a ruler and a map grid to figure out how far we would go. I take full responsibility in any inaccuracies and beg your forgiveness as these are supposed to be representative.

Some of these routes were chosen because they touched a very special part of me for different reasons. These biblical journeys represent different themes to me and I will share with you how they became a part of the Christ Walk journey.

The first year I did Christ Walk, I think I had only three different routes to choose from: a beginner route, an intermediate route, and an advanced route to challenge different fitness levels. Over the years, I have added other routes as I journeyed through the Bible. I have also added "group routes" because we are all in this together! Research supports the positive impact of groups and teamwork on success in obtaining goals. People who set goals together are more likely to stick with them and be successful.

The Nazareth Challenge   This was one of the first routes I developed. It is 60 miles between Jesus' hometown of Nazareth and Jerusalem. This is approximately 1.6 miles each day for forty days to walk the distance of the route that Jesus preached to reach Jerusalem. The goal was very special to me because as a military wife, I am often far from home. I look at my journey now as leading me to my final resting spot one day and I find that very satisfying.

The Jerusalem to Damascus Route   This journey represents Paul's conversion on the Damascus Road. The route is approximately 3.75 miles per day. What an amazing journey to find your way as a Christian and growing in God's love. I can think of no greater journey than Paul's conversion. If he could walk this route blind, anyone can do it. For me personally, I have a hearing loss that I will tell you more about in another chapter, but Paul's loss of eyesight did not stop him from his calling. This is a wonderful journey to choose.

The Jerusalem Challenge   During Jesus' final days, his route through Jerusalem included preaching at the temple, the clearing of the temple, his last meal with his disciples, his arrest at Gethsemane, his trial, Peter's denial, and then his crucifixion on Golgotha. This route is roughly 2.2 miles per day. This is known as the *Via Dolorosa* or The Way of Suffering. What a powerful image to walk the distance of Christ's ultimate sacrifice for us each day. You can reflect as you walk on this great gift we have been given. This is a lovely, lovely journey to try as you explore your spirituality and relationship to God. Can you walk a day in Jesus' shoes? Can you walk forty days in Jesus' shoes? If so, this is the route for you to tackle.

The Damascus to Caesarea Journey   This is a journey of 5 miles a day representing the walks that the disciples took on their missionary journeys. I find it inspiring that the disciples traveled such great distances without cars or other forms of modern transportation. Aside from a donkey or camel, these journeys were taken by foot. See yourself as part of that missionary journey and step proudly each day on your challenge. Look at this challenge as a physical testament to your belief in God.

The Bethlehem Challenge   I think of this challenge as the Alpha and Omega Challenge. It is about 5 miles between Bethlehem and Jerusalem and represents walking the route from Jesus' birth to his death. This *is* Jesus' journey from where God put him in the world to his ultimate calling. Where will your journey take you?

The Exodus Challenge   Not for the faint of heart, this challenge was chosen for some of the most advanced of my Christ Walk participants. This is the route the Jews traveled to get to the Promised Land: 375 miles or 9.4 miles per day or 18,750 steps per day (you may also use this one as a group challenge). We are all on our journey to the Promised Land.

Appendix A in the book have additional group journeys where teams can pool their miles towards additional (and longer) routes found in the Bible. The second year I did Christ Walk, I learned that the journey was a lot more fun when we did it with teams. The teams provided a support system to get each of us through our different strengths and weakness on our routes.

If you are doing Christ Walk as a group, I recommend that during the first week, you arrange for some fitness professionals to come in and discuss principles of healthy living. It is useful to have them provide some type of fitness testing so that you can receive baseline information on the fitness level of your body. These evaluations, such as blood pressure, resting heart rate, body mass index, weight, and cardiovascular fitness can give you some objective information on what you need to change or improve. These tests can be repeated at the end of the journey to show the progress you have made.

There may be another route that speaks more deeply to you than these favorites of mine, and I encourage you to find that route and take it. I have always let the Christ Walk participants find their own journeys. The point is to get up and get moving. You cannot start the journey if you are sitting down.

Each day, there will be a place for you to fill in your steps/distance, your activity, your feelings for the day, and your spiritual thought for the day. Do not rush to finish the book. This book is designed to be read one chapter a day, as a journal to help you on your way and improve your Christ Walk experience. If at any time you need to change your goals, feel free to do so. Life is a journey with many bumps happening along the way! The challenge is that you continue to have faith to continue on the journey, even if it is in a different way than the one in which you started. If you are doing this as a group, these journal entries may help your group to share their Christ Walk experience and deepen your understanding of a life of walking with Christ. See Appendix D for Suggestions for Groups.

So, how do we measure the steps we took, the distance we traveled? I recommend the purchase of a pedometer or fitness tracker, which can be clipped to your belt or pants and will track the number of steps/miles traveled each day. Recommendations from the experts encourage every individual to take 10,000 steps a day for heart health. You may need to work up to this level of activity, and perhaps this will be one of your goals. Roughly 2,000 to 2,500 steps equal a mile. Depending on the type of pedometer, it may tell you this, or you may have to calculate your stride if you want to be more accurate. For the purpose of Christ Walk, we generally give one mile for every 2,000 steps. There is a brief description of using a pedometer in Appendix B.

If you want to use another form of exercise other than walking (biking, swimming, aerobics, dance, etc.) you may do that. It takes about fifteen minutes to walk a mile, so every fifteen-minute block of exercise can be calculated as a "mile." The important thing is to choose an activity that you enjoy and do it. The purpose is to get out there and move, to think about every activity you do as walking with God. It is your walk with Christ, so you will have to take it up with your conscience if you cheat! Your job is to give it your best shot with all your heart.

Mileage Calculation Chart

Activity	Time	Steps	Record Miles As:
Walking	15–20 minutes	2,000–2,500	1 or distance on route
Running	Varies	2,000–2,500	Check route distance
Biking	Varies	N/A	Check odometer distance
Aerobics	15 minutes	Varies	1
Dancing	15 minutes	Varies	1
Yoga	15 minutes	Varies	1
Prayer/Meditation	15 minutes	Varies	1
Volunteerism	15 minutes	Varies	1

Take your first step(s) and see how many steps your pedometer took you today. Set a goal to add more steps each day to your journey to work up to 10,000 steps a day in whatever activity you choose.

THOUGHTS TO PONDER

1. What is my goal?

2. How do I feel about my goal? Is it reasonable/attainable/realistic?
If not, how can I make it something that I will stick with for the next
forty days?

3. Who can help me on my journey?

*Surely the land on which your foot has trodden shall be an inheritance for you
and your children forever, because you have wholeheartedly followed the Lord
my God.* —Joshua 14:9

DAY 1 Steps taken: 12,062   Miles journeyed: 5.05

Exercise chosen: Walking

Spiritual thoughts: Jesus did all that Walking in Jesus sandals. They don't look very comfortable.

Feelings: My shins hurt. My little bird-like feet bones hurt. It took much longer to walk 1 mile than it should. I will improve.

Using a Pedometer

BIBLICAL BIG IDEA #2

Teach them to your children, talking about them when you are at home and when you are away, when you lie down and when you rise. —Deuteronomy 11:19

A pedometer or fitness tracker is a nifty little tool that counts each step you take. We use the pedometer as an easy tool to track all the steps we take in our walk with Christ each day. The pedometer is not there to be a jockey whipping a horse towards the finish line; rather it is there to give you guideposts on how far you have gone toward the goals that you have set. You will get more comfortable with the pedometer the more you use it. Strap it on and take it for a whirl for a couple of days to find out how far you go in an average day. The minimum recommendation is 10,000 steps a day for heart health.

So how far did you go with your pedometer? Were you able to reach 10,000 steps? Did you fall short? That is okay. Falling short is all about being human. The trick is to pray about it and get up the next day and try again. I think every time a human tries a little harder, God smiles. If you are so far off 10,000 steps that you do not think you can commit to Christ Walk, I pray that you consider doing incremental goals. There are ways to "sneak" in extra steps to your day such as taking the stairs, parking at the back of a parking lot, walking to work or shopping or school. Consider taking three ten-minute walks instead of one thirty-minute one and then gradually increasing as your endurance and enjoyment of the activity increases.

If you are walking 4,000–5,000 steps each day (which, by the way, is the average American movement in one day), please set a weekly goal of increasing your steps by 2,000 steps a day for a couple of weeks until you reach the goal of walking 10,000 steps per day. You do not have to start out with 10,000 steps if this is new to you. Gradually build up towards this goal. If by the end of the forty days you have trained yourself to walk 10,000 steps a day, you have made a marvelous transformation. Perhaps your next forty-day Christ Walk will be to complete one of the routes. And perhaps the one after that will be to go a longer route. Your Christ Walk is only as short as you limit yourself. If you never stop walking with Christ, then you never stop your Christ Walk.

While I again stress that this is NOT a diet or weight-loss program, I do want to caution you that 10,000 steps a day is the minimum requirement for cardiovascular health. That is heart health. That is how well your ticker keeps ticking. I am a big believer that I want my ticker to go as strong and hard as it can. I would like to maintain a level of high physical fitness as long as possible so that I can continue to do what I am called to do. If I do not take care of my heart, it is certainly not going to take care of me. I pray often that I am able to stay active and healthy and walking until I am finally called by God.

There is a difference between cardiovascular health and weight loss. Most individuals who use a pedometer for weight loss will have to log 12,000–15,000 steps each day. They also have to watch what they eat. We will discuss food (and how much I love food) in a later chapter. But be advised as you start your goals and revise them that there may be more steps needed to meet whatever goals you set for yourself. Ten thousand steps a day is the minimum for which to strive.

While we do focus on steps per day as a part of Christ Walk, because of the analogy of physically walking with Christ, you do not have to be limited by walking. Walking is simply the most popular form of exercise, the easiest to do, and the one exercise that people are most likely to stick with over time. I enjoy running, sometimes. I like biking, sometimes. I like walking a lot of the time. I like swimming, sometimes. I like aerobic classes, sometimes, and I like weight lifting a lot. I want to write, "Pick your poison," but that has a negative connotation. What I want you to do is pick something and do it. And if you have to pick a lot of "somethings," that is okay as well. The point is to think about getting up and doing. Our bodies were designed to move. Whatever you want to do, get up and do it.

Remember, every fifteen-minute block of physical activity is worth one mile towards your goal, or if you bike, run, swim, etc. faster than a mile in fifteen minutes, log the actual miles! Just move and log that distance.

I am married to a lawyer, so of course I must insert the disclaimer that if you have never before exercised or set such a goal for yourself, please discuss your plans with your healthcare provider to ensure that your physical safety is addressed. These professionals are goldmines of health information and can be a partner on your journey if you ask! Develop a relationship with your healthcare provider and do not take "no" for an answer. Pursue him or her until you get the information you need. If you are worried that your physical health will keep you from your journey, do not fear: I have had individuals with walkers and wheelchairs participate in the Christ Walk journey. Your trail is only limited by your imagination. Faith in God will keep you going along the way.

Mental and spiritual nourishment are also very important to your journey. For every fifteen-minute period of time that you are using to nourish your spirit and mind, log yourself a mile! Research has shown that people who meditate and pray have lower blood pressure and feelings of stress. This is all good towards taking care of the temple. So take credit for it! We also Christ Walk when we do for others. Volunteering is a great way to get bonus steps and every fifteen minutes of volunteering is worth another mile. My only caveat is that this is designed for us to move and walk and think about our Christ Walk daily. I encourage you to spend most of your miles in moving each day.

And when in doubt about how to move or what to do, pray.

THOUGHTS TO PONDER

1. Were you able to start walking or Christ Walking as you had hoped?

2. If not, what were your barriers? Do you need help overcoming the barriers? Who can help you?

3. Did you feel rejuvenated by the experience of starting a new journey? If so, write it down, so it will help motivate you along the way.

All things can be done for the one who believes. —Mark 9:23

DAY 2 Steps taken: 12,859 Miles journeyed: 5.42

Exercise chosen: Walk

Spiritual thoughts: Took a new route, good to see new things

Feelings: Still slow. I hope to increase my pace. Sore again today, and feel blister coming on bottom of my foot

How We Are Created

BIBLICAL BIG IDEA #3

So God created humankind in his image, in the image of God he created them; male and female he created them.
—Genesis 1:27

Let me tell you about the temple. We are the temple for God's work in the world. Jesus, the Word of God, was with God, and therefore he has been with us since the beginning. He came to earth to reconcile our sins and bridge the gap between God and humans. Jesus is the living covenant of God's relationship with us. Through Jesus, we have a wonderful opportunity for a relationship with God. And I believe that the Holy Spirit dwells within each of us.

Do you not know that your body is a temple of the Holy Spirit within you, which you have from God, and that you are not your own? For you were bought with a price; therefore glorify God in your body. —1 Corinthians 6:19–20

This is the God-spark we all have that calls us to do great things in the world. And therefore, our bodies are our temples. I feel called to take care of that temple so that the God-spark in me has a great place to live and do its work in the world. If I do not take care of the temple, the God-spark has nowhere to do its work in the world.

It is not about being skinny. I look around me and see beautiful people. They come in all shapes and sizes, all colors, all different elasticity, all different fitness levels. We are all creatures of God. We are all made in God's image. Therefore, there is diversity in how we all look, but that does not make any of us less beautiful than the other. We are all amazingly beautiful.

If you started this program as a diet or weight-loss program, I pray that you reconsider. Christ Walk is about a type of living—Christ-centered living—wherever we walk and whatever we do is done for the glory of God. Our bodies were made to move and to do things. We are designed to pray, create, live joyfully, be giving, and be active. I have struggled for years with the conflict between what secular society tells me I am supposed to look like as a woman and letting go, tuning out secular society to hear that God loves me as I am. That God made me, as I am, and it is my choice to do with the gifts God gave me. When I use those gifts to God's glory, I am living in Christ Walk. I have turned from what people say I should look like, and have turned to the way God has made me and realized that I am beautiful—that we are all beautiful—as we are made. There are a lot of miserable people in the world that are striving for a perfection that they will never get, because they are not God. My joy comes not from how others perceive I look, but rather the joy that I get from doing the right thing and using the gift of my body towards God's will.

You may feel that I am talking out of two sides of my mouth. How can we have a program that is designed to build healthy individuals, mind, body, and soul, but is not about a diet, nor the way we look? It is not about your perception of yourself, or others' perception of you; it is about what your temple can do to glorify God.

Do not be driven by worries about what others think; worry about what God thinks.

A couple of years ago I decided to run a half marathon. I was doing this to lose weight. I struggled with my weight, or rather, I struggled mentally with what I thought was a healthy weight in terms of what the magazines say. Now I have come to realize that my healthy weight is where I feel comfortable in my skin.

However, I did need to lose some weight after having my second child, so I decided to run. I had never run before. I never really did like running, and I sure felt like every step I took was a showcase of everything wrong with me bobbling about on the track. But I started the whole training program focused on me: obsessing about what was wrong with me, obsessing about my speed, and obsessing about what people were thinking as they watched me struggle to run. And I was miserable. I hated every moment of the run. My thoughts became self-defeating repetitions that caused me to stop, stumble, and want to give up.

Then one day, God spoke to me on my run. I believe I was crying at the time about how much I hated to run when I heard, "Don't do it for you." Huh? Whodathunk? And so I started to pick up speed, gained a little more confidence, and started to hatch a plan that I would not run for myself, but that I would find something that meant something more than me to run for. And so, I ran home just as fast as you please and bold as brass told my husband and my neighbor upstairs (who also went to church with us) that they were going to train and run a local half marathon with me; we were going to raise money for the local mission team as a part of it.

This was a part of Christ Walk IV at Emmanuel Episcopal Church. I knew that I needed to take the program to the next step. We needed a new focus after four years of the program and this was it. In six weeks we raised over $3,500 for the next mission trip just through word of mouth. I felt GREAT! Every time I thought I might stumble on my run, I prayed to God that he would hold me up because this wasn't about me anymore. I had a reason to run. Something that was bigger and better than anything I could do and I felt good. I was using my body for the glory of God.

During the race itself, I remember getting to mile 9.5 and starting to feel weak. It is *hard* to run. I do not know how athletes do it over and over again. I do like running, but it will never be easy. When I got weak, I prayed. I prayed for God's strength to wrap around my legs and get me home and it did. And it was exhilarating! God is great. With God you can do anything.

This is an example of taking care of the temple. You can run and improve your body and work it to take care of God's work in the world. You can look at bad habits and change them for a healthier you and still be doing this for God's vision of you in the world. Just don't expect that God's vision of you is to be movie-star thin or whatever flavor of the month is "in."

I do not believe that God intended for us to be miserable in our own skin. God made us in a lot of different ways and we need to put aside what society says we need to look like and focus on loving what we can do for our bodies, with our bodies, and for other bodies.

THOUGHTS TO PONDER

1. How do you feel about you in your own skin? Is it a healthy vision of you? Does it feel *right* with what you know about God's vision for you?

2. What do you think society says about you? How can you reconcile secular beliefs with your belief in God?

Do you not know that your body is a temple of the Holy Spirit within you, which you have from God, and that you are not your own? For you were bought with a price; therefore glorify God in your body. —1 Corinthians 6:19–20

DAY 3 Steps taken: 10,400   Miles journeyed: 4.35

Exercise chosen: eliptical, cleaning up fallen tree

Spiritual thoughts: Plans change, go w/ the flow

Feelings: I had planned to exercise more 4 Eric, but he came here and our tree had fallen on our neighbors driveway, so we had to clean it up. Good exercise.

4 Types of Walking

BIBLICAL BIG IDEA #4

You must follow exactly the path that the LORD your God has commanded you, so that you may live, and that it may go well with you, and that you may live long in the land that you are to possess. —Deuteronomy 5:33

Did you know that there are different ways to walk? We can stroll, we can move with purpose, we can hike; we can do all sorts of things. Walking can be broken down into leisure walking, fitness walking, and speed walking. You can also look at walking as walking with God (meditative walking), walking with friends (communal walking), and walking alone—although you really are not alone, because God is always with you on your walks.

Leisure walking is just as it sounds: walking for the pleasure of walking. It is great for the body, good for the knees, good for the environment (walking cuts down on the use of cars and gasoline emissions in the community, thereby decreasing pollution), and a great way to be outdoors and enjoy where you live. Leisure walking is walking for the fun of walking. One of the things that I absolutely adored about my time living in Germany was that Sundays were still Holy Days. By law, no businesses were open. Many Germans, while not practicing Christians, had a day of rest. My husband and I called Sundays "walking days" because on Sunday, after a leisurely morning and long lunch, the Germans walked. They walked on most days of the week, but on Sunday everyone was out walking or biking. They did not go to stores, or movies, or conduct business. They went out as family and friends and walked.

I recently heard a discussion about how Americans have forgotten to have a day of rest. Even with going to church, Sundays have become the day to catch up on everything else because we are too busy being busy. This is a shame for a number of reasons. One, our bodies need rest. Two, the Lord directed us to have a day of rest. And three, when was the last time we just went out and enjoyed being out, walking with our families for the enjoyment of spending time together? If I had a wish, it is that we could bring back walking Sundays and days of rest without business or bustle. Consider making Sunday your walking day, your family day, or your rest day. Leave the housework, yard work, the shopping for another day. They will be there waiting for you; your family may not.

Fitness walking is the next type of walking. It is actually a different kind of walking that calls for you to center yourself in your core (your core is your midsection—I had a trainer tell me to think of your belly button kissing your spine, and this has stuck with me as a great visual for engaging your core). You will need to stand up straight, elbows bent at a 90-degree angle, and walk briskly, heel to toe, while swinging your arms. It is incredibly difficult to describe with words. Part of it is taking your leisure walk, standing up straight, and taking off faster. A fitness walk is about three to four miles an hour and your heart should be beating fast enough that you feel the effort of the exercise. You should feel as though you are getting a workout. You should find it slightly difficult to talk while walking.

Speed walking is a very fast walk that is over four miles an hour. The form for a speed walk is to walk at a VERY fast pace with your body tilted slightly forward and powering through the balls of your feet and toes. Your hips move side to side a little more with speed walking. I have a friend who speed walks, and let us just say that she can walk faster than I can run. It also helps that she has the legs of an Amazon. She hates to run, but loves to walk. She is amazing.

Just as there are different types of walking, there are also different types of running, different types of biking, and different types of any other exercise you may do. There are different levels of training with exercises because there are different levels of athleticism. I am not an athlete. Athletes think very differently about the body and exercise than I do. I am happy to keep my heart going and my feet moving. That would not be the way an athlete thought about his or her body. This is okay. God created athletes, ultra-athletes, professional athletes, performance athletes, fitness gurus, and everyday Joes and Jills who want to stay healthy. God created us all: we are more than the Baskin Robbins 31 flavors. There are many more flavors of God's creation.

Just as there are different types of exercise and different levels of athleticism, there are different types of bodies. We all have different types of bodies. The point is to take care of our bodies. We are made in the image of God—ALL of us—not just the athletes, or the models, or the actors. God made the moms, the dads, the teenagers, the babies, the workers, the handicapped—*all* of us. That means we need to take care of how God made us. Sometimes that means moving more. Sometimes that means not filling the hole in our hearts with unnecessary food. Sometimes that means doing more for others, but it's all about Christ Walking.

Whatever walking you choose, I pray that you consider opening your mind to God's voice during this time. Some of my best prayer time comes during walking as I have left the distractions of home and hearth and work behind. I allow my mind to talk to God to discuss things that are great, things that are good, and things that are not so good, and also to listen to God. A relationship with God is all about sharing and talking to God. It does not have to be a formal prayer, or specific rote words. Rather, it is about talking to God and then LISTENING.

The idea for Christ Walk came to me on a walk. I had worked with walking programs through my job but I needed to do something with the church that I felt called to do. I am not much of a Sunday school teacher, I tend to be too opinionated for the vestry, but I knew I was passionate about health and spirituality and that I could do something with this. I heard God call me because I took the time to listen.

You would think it sounds like I have it down with my relationship with God and my prayer life and my listening life. But I don't. I mess up a lot. I know when I have gotten it right, and I know when I have gotten it wrong. I am very human, very flawed, but filled with the grace and forgiveness of God.

God's call keeps knocking on my door and saying, "Just do it," no matter how unequipped I may feel to finish the job. But when I am walking, God is helping me through my concerns and questions. God is giving me guidance on where to go. When I find God's peace on my walk, that's when I know I am doing it right.

THOUGHTS TO PONDER

1. How is your walk? Or your other fitness goal, if you have chosen something other than walking?

2. Are you praying? Have you heard God on your walks? If so, what did he say?

3. What do you need to do to "Just do it" ?

They heard the sound of the Lord *God walking in the garden at the time of the evening breeze, and the man and his wife hid themselves from the presence of the* Lord *God among the trees of the garden.* —Genesis 3:8–9

DAY 4   Steps taken: *8769*   Miles journeyed: *3.67*

Exercise chosen: *Small walk, eliptical*

Spiritual thoughts: _____

_____

_____

_____

Feelings: *Fitbit doesn't trach*
Eliptical, so hopefully I
walked more than calculated

_____

_____

DAY 5 Journeys in the Bible

BIBLICAL BIG IDEA #5

Go in peace. The mission you are on is under the eye of the LORD. —Judges 18:6

Why are we here? God created us with a purpose. We have a journey to take during our time here on earth. We are not here for ourselves. I believe that many people have great dissatisfaction in their lives because they are so focused on themselves and *their* needs. We took the concept of "me time," which is not necessarily a bad thing, but turned it into "me *all* the time." When I realized that my purpose was not about myself, but God, I felt relieved. It was an amazing gift to hear that. I felt like a burden had been lifted from my shoulders when I discovered, "It's not about you."

If it's not about me, then we were created with purpose to do for others. If you let go of the burden of what society, government, politics, movies, magazines, and others try to tell you is your purpose and rather focus on what you feel called to do for your family, friends, church, and community, then I think you will find the burden lifted from your shoulders. There is such great joy in letting go of the self and doing for others. As I discussed in the previous chapter, my journey for health frustrated me until I included others in my goal and made my running about doing for others, not just for myself.

I therefore, the prisoner in the Lord, beg you to lead a life worthy of the calling to which you have been called. —Ephesians 4:1

Live a life that is called for service to others, not as a slave to what society is directing.

Here is a little exercise for you: Get a piece of paper. I like a 3 x 5 card because I can fold it and keep it in my wallet as a reminder. Think about something you either want to change about yourself or something you've always wanted to do but have been afraid to do. Write it on one side of your card. On the other side, write the three most important things in your life.

For me, the three most important things are God, my family, and my health. These may be yours as well. Many people have God and family in the top three; sometimes a job is also considered important. When you look back at what you want to change about yourself, is it reflected in the three most important things in your life? How can you use the three most important things to help you?

For example, if you need to quit smoking and you cannot find the strength to do it, consider that smoking does not support the most important things in your life: It may take time away from your devotion to God; it is an addiction (one that costs money and has great impacts for you, your family, and the environment). Smoking is terrible for your health. This thing about yourself that you want to change is rarely supported by the three most important things in your life.

If you are addicted to tobacco, food, drink, drugs, or whatever it may be you have given so much of your vital energy to an inanimate thing that takes you away from your time with God and your family; and it is probably bad for your health. God would rather you be addicted to him than addicted to a vice. And God can give you the power to overcome that vice.

Consider your family. Tobacco, or whatever other bad habit you may want to address, has physical ramifications for your family. Children of smokers have multiple health problems. These habits cost a great deal of money, which could be a burden on your family. The toxins are damaging to your home, and your family would be utterly lost without you if you were to die from your habit. Needless to say, if health was one of your most important priorities, tobacco use or ANY other addiction is bad for your health. I hope that goes without saying.

I also hope that you see this exercise as a positive reinforcement for *why* you can change your life. You have three important things to lift you up and take on any challenge or goal that you may have. You have three important things that give you purpose in this life. You have three important things that you can use in building your devotion and relationship with God. I used this exercise in helping me to get going with this book. I knew I needed to write this book, but it was much harder than I ever thought it could be. I knew also that writing this book supported the three most important things in my life. I used this exercise to quit smoking myself. I used this exercise when I needed to reexamine my nutritional habits and focus on what supported what I said was important in my life. You can do this too.

I hope that you see that the three most important things in your life are an important part of your journey. Your journey here on earth was ordained by God. I do not believe that we live a meaningless existence here at the whim of a petulant God. I believe that God is revealed to all of us at different points in our lives and in different ways. If we focus on the important things in our life, everything else will come together on the journey.

THOUGHTS TO PONDER

1. Is there something I want to change about myself or work towards?

2. What are the three most important things in my life?

3. What are three things that are keeping me from being successful with my goal?

4. What can I do to overcome them?

Consider the ravens: they neither sow nor reap, they have neither storehouse nor barn, and yet God feeds them. Of how much more value are you than the birds! —Luke 12:24

DAY 5 Steps taken: _8994_ Miles journeyed: _3.76_

Exercise chosen: _Eliptical_

Spiritual thoughts: _Maybe I need a day of no cookies (baking, decorating, etc) whatsoever. Need to focus on other things. Hard to do tho, lots of orders_

Feelings: _It rained all day, so walking wasn't an option. 2 miles on the eliptical barely register on the Fitbit which is discouraging_

DAY 6 The Mind, Body, and Spirit Connection

BIBLICAL BIG IDEA #6

You shall love the Lord your God with all your heart, and with all your soul, and with all your mind. —Matthew 22:37

Research supports the notion that mind, body, and spiritual health are all connected. In fact, the World Health Organization's definition of health is a state of "complete physical, mental, and social well-being and not merely the absence of disease or infirmity." This definition has not changed since 1948. As a Christian, I believe, and a great deal of research supports, that spiritual well-being is essential for physical and mental health. When we are not "right" with our spirit, our bodies and minds can fail. Spiritual illnesses can cause great mental pain and anguish. Similarly, physical and mental infirmity can cause a strain on the spirit. There are stories of people whose doctors could find nothing physically wrong with a patient and yet they continued to fail in their well-being because their spirit was so ill.

Conversely, strong mental, spiritual, and/or physical health can help you overcome disease and illness of the mind or body when they are threatened. Taking care of your mind, body, and spirit is *good* for the mind, body, and spirit. When Jesus heals the paralytic in Luke 5:17–26, Jesus first has to heal the man's spirit before he can heal his body. Jesus drove evil spirits from minds and souls in order to heal. Jesus knew that these individuals must be reconciled with him in order to attain the healing they sought. Faith has healed many people.

If we look back on our discussion about the things we want to change about ourselves, these things (smoking, drinking, food, stress, etc.) are our addictions and vices. We often turn to these things before turning to God in order to cope. We look for solace in food or alcohol or drugs in an attempt to manage our spiritual, mental, or physical distress, thereby compounding our problems. Before we can become strong physically, we often need to address these addictions and seek help in putting them behind us. If we replace our addictions with a God-centered life, then we are capable of accomplishing so much with our physical wellbeing. Like the transformation of the water into wine at the wedding of Cana, we have an opportunity to allow Jesus to transform us into so much more if we allow God into our life.

I smoked back in college. I was a nursing student and smoked. If I could have had a big fat "idiot" label plastered across my forehead, I had it, even if I did not see it. The smoking started after a bad breakup. Then with the stress of school ending and as the impending independence from my parents began to loom, my smoking habit got worse. It seemed like a harmless way to deal with the stress in my life. I also felt very cool and mature. Then I met my future husband and he was none-too-pleased with my nasty habit, so I started the journey to quit. I knew intellectually, thanks to four years of nursing school, that tobacco use is a terrible habit. Even though I was not a heavy smoker, nor did I use cigarettes for an extended length of time, I found smoking incredibly addictive. Tobacco is an addictive drug. It stimulates a satisfaction center in the brain. It is also considered a gateway drug, as it reduces inhibitions to trying other risky behaviors, including excessive drinking or drug use. The number one habit to break in support of a healthier life is using tobacco products.

Although I quit smoking, I found the stress of a patient dying on the ward would send me back to sneaking a smoke on a break with the other nurses. Then I would feel guilty and try to hide it from my husband. This was a short but vicious cycle until I thought about my three most important things. This habit was keeping me from my relationship with God. I could have chosen to talk to God about my stress, my anxiety, my problems, and my grief, but it was a lot easier for me to turn to a smoke. It was terrible to my health and the fact I tried to hide it from my family was just plain wrong. There was nothing about my habit that was supporting the three most important things in my life.

In order to finally quit smoking for good, I turned to God in prayer and prayed that he would give me the strength to overcome this habit. I prayed that my desire for the nicotine would be banished. I have never smoked since. I have felt no desire for cigarettes since that time. I give thanks to God for the strength he gave me. I have learned to replace my bad habits with healthier habits of prayer, physical exercise, and mental exercise. These healthy habits of prayer, exercise, good nutrition, and meditation are the prescription for many unhealthy habits. You need to arm yourself with the tools for success.

We will talk more about additional tools to success as we go through the chapters. But do not doubt that you can be successful. I know you can and God knows you can. Don't be the one to say, "I can't."

You have the Christ-spark inside you. What a precious thing we all carry! As a mother, I think of my Christ-spark like the child I carried in my womb for nine months. We all have this spark and we can joyfully nurture this spark. We are the temple of this Christ-spark. We need to take care of its temple so that it can do marvelous things in the world.

"Before I formed you in the womb I knew you, and before you were born I consecrated you; I appointed you a prophet to the nations." —Jeremiah 1:5

God has a purpose for every person. And every purpose when fulfilled to the glory of God is a good thing. Connect your spiritual and physical health so that you are nurturing both. Then your health choices will be focused on both spiritual and physical fitness.

THOUGHTS TO PONDER

1. What is your purpose right now at this point in your life?

2. Has your purpose changed? Do you think it will change in the future?

3. How does your purpose make you feel?

4. Do you think you need to rethink your purpose to ensure the three most important things in your life are a part of it?

I know that you can do all things, and that no purpose of yours can be thwarted. —Job 42:2

DAY 6 Steps taken: _13,098_ Miles journeyed: _5.6_

Exercise chosen: _Walk_

Spiritual thoughts: _Not supposed to focus on_
the # on the scale, but need
motivation

Feelings: _My scale is not cooperating._
Getting a new one today

So what does the world of health look like? What does health look like when it is created in God's eyes? Health is harmony of the mind, body, and spirit towards God's will. Health feels good. It smells good, it tastes good, it sounds good, and it looks good. We know what it is like to have health. We also know what it is like not to have health. Health can be very hard for some people to obtain. When we were given the freedom to make choices, the implications of those choices are often played out in our health and the health of generations to come.

Health is not defined by society. What may be healthy for one individual may be a different level of health for another. Many societal ideas on "health" can actually be unhealthy. Health is not solely defined by the absence of disease. Having infirmity does not necessarily mean you are not healthy. Health is different for different people at different points in time. Health is not the status quo or stagnant. Levels of health change throughout one's life. Loss of a health level can be devastating, but improvements in health can be an amazing experience. Sometimes we need to have a health shock before we realize we are not as healthy as we thought we were.

We are told from so many directions what health is and what we should be doing for our health. Sometimes everything we are doing or should be doing gets a little overwhelming and can also make us unhealthy with worry. We have forgotten how to know ourselves and our balances and to align our mind, body, and spirit. Sometimes we have to make decisions about our health that feel right to our gut, but fly in the face of conventional wisdom. This is okay. This can be healthy too.

Our bodies were meant to move. When we do not take care of our bodies, we cannot do the work we are called to do: as mother, father, sister, brother, son, daughter, coworker, church member, colleague, leader, or follower. Because so much of the activity in our lives has been taken over by technology, we need to figure out how to move our bodies to God's will in order to keep the body doing God's work in the world.

It is easy to blame God when health fails. Disease is not of God. God is with us through our illnesses. Sometimes it doesn't make sense when health fails, especially in small children or otherwise healthy adults. Changes in societal health choices such as environmental impacts, technology, food and water sources, medications, and others can have long-ranging impacts across generations of which we may be unaware. God will comfort us through these times.

The good news is that we do have the tools and the gifts from God to get back on track. Health of mind, body, and spirit should be celebrated. I often think of our life as a journey. I believe that our reason here on earth is ordained, because we have a purpose and a reason for being here. Each of us goes out in the world as a representative of God's love to one another. Each step we take on this journey is fulfilling our calling to God. This is our gift to our community at large. The Christian tradition supports a healthy life. Christ Walk supports this Christian tradition through healthy choices towards physical exercise, eating, prayer, and education. God will support us and strengthen us through all these choices so we are creating a healthy life with God.

PART TWO

SIN

DAY
7 Stress

BIBLICAL BIG IDEA #7:

To set the mind on the flesh is death, but to set the mind on the Spirit is life and peace. —Romans 8:6

Stress kills. Well, bad stress can kill. Stress that is not channelled creatively or through activity causes negative biofeedback patterns that result in an elevated heart rate, increased blood pressure, and changes in hormone levels. These changes can affect every part of the body through the vast network of neural paths and the lymphatic system.

I find it ironic that, with all the conveniences of modern-day living, we work harder than ever. Instead of clearing time in our lives for family and prayer, technology has created a heightened level of stress and need for more work. We no longer work in tune with the changing of the seasons. Instead we force our bodies to work against our normal circadian rhythms and at longer hours than ever before. The standard "forty-hour work week" really is not so. The hours of overtime and stress associated with our jobs have come at the expense of our health. Compounded with that, the very technology that makes some parts of our lives easier is bad for our health. We move less now because so many machines do the physical labor for us.

It is easier to get our food, but unfortunately, so much food has unnecessary processing done to it that it is less healthy food. Today's food has so many "modern-day additives" that we don't know the effect these foods are having on our bodies. I cannot tell you the number of times I have picked up an "all natural" food to find it really has a number of additives and preservatives. Foods are genetically modified now and we really do not know the impact of these foods on our bodies or to future generations. We do not know what we are doing to the world for future generations. But, unfortunately, when we start messing around with how things are made genetically, I believe that can cause a big problem somewhere down the line. Perhaps it is my ignorance, but I fail to see how we can improve on the bounty available to us in God's good earth.

Technology can be a very good thing. My computer makes writing incredibly easy. My hearing aids have allowed me to hear again. My vacuum helps me clean, as do my other appliances. Despite all these technological conveniences, we continue to stress. The problem with bad stress is that it leads to sin. This type of stress is like another gateway drug to addictive behaviors, behaviors that can lead us to sin. Sin to me is when we are separated from God. When we cease to converse with God, we sin. Stress has a tendency to keep us from communicating with God. In fact, the more stress we have, the more it distracts us from talking it over with God and working the issues through in a Christian manner. And when we are not talking to God, we are more likely to snap at our family, friends, colleagues, and self in a way that is not kind, nor Christ-like.

I know that when I am stressed, my inclination is to take the stance, "I'm not going to bother God with this; this is too small, too petty, and he's got bigger things to worry about." I have sinned, because 1) I quit talking to God, 2) tried to put a size on God and, 3) I made a big, fat assumption about God's capabilities that isn't even close to the truth.

So stress is bad for your relationship with God, it's bad for your health, and it's probably bad for your family too. I don't think stress fits into the top three things in my life!

Anxiety weighs down the human heart. —Proverbs 12:25a

But stress doesn't go away. In fact, sometimes when we are trying our hardest to stay focused and Christ-centered, it seems that there are even more stressful situations being thrown at us.

Sometimes the attempt to find the right physical exercise and the right foods can cause stress. For example, I find going to the grocery store stressful because there are so many choices. When I think I am making healthy choices, I discover that there are so many hidden things in food to make it an unhealthy choice. It is exhausting and stressful! Often, when we are wrapped up in trying to do the "right thing" and act the "right way," we forget to put God in the center of our decisions. When we separate God from the times we are trying to do the right thing and make the right decision, we can experience stress. When we separate God from ourselves, in even the small decisions and choices, we have chosen to sin. God should be with us in all decisions, both big and small. This will help to reduce stress in our lives.

I encourage you not to give up. Put God back in the middle of the stress. Put God in the beginning of all your decisions. The best things for dealing with a stressful, or stress-filled, life are to pray, exercise, and eat right.

God should be a part of all of this. When you support the mind, body, and spirit connection you can offset the effects of the stress in your life. It is well documented how meditation and prayer reduces heart rate and blood pressure while increasing cardio-pulmonary perfusion. In layman's terms, this means that the blood vessels in the body relax so that blood flows to the vital organs (like the heart, lungs, and brain) more efficiently, which allows for a greater percentage of oxygen to reach all parts of the body. Exercise releases endorphins (feel-good hormones) that offset the cortico-steroids (stress hormones) released during the stressful situation. A healthy diet filled with wholesome, real, nutritious food (real food is food from the earth and the creatures that God gave us) can help block the effects of free-radicals and stress chemicals introduced to the body. Exercise and a healthy diet keep the system clean and improve the immune system so that you do not get sick from the stress. Exercise and healthy eating also continue to build the strength of your temple, your body.

Continuing the temple analogy from Day One, if there are cracks and fissures in your temple, stress helps to widen those cracks and cause the temple to fail. Stress is also a gateway to picking up really bad habits, including alcohol or drug abuse, mindless eating, and a sedentary life. Stress can fill your mind so that you cannot clear it to focus on prayer and worship, and stress can tangle your tongue when communicating with friends in which harsh words can ensue. Bad stress can bring out the very worst in us. If we can channel the energy created by stressful environments into a positive outlet, some wonderful creative moments can occur.

Positive ways to channel stress can include:

- Prayer
- Exercise
- Cooking
- Painting
- Writing
- Meditation
- Singing
- Music
- Woodwork
- Play
- Projects
- Support groups/friends/relationship building
- Art

Create several outlets for yourself to channel your stress whether at work or at home in order to have an immediate way to deal with stress and have an outlet for overall stress throughout your life.

Cast all your anxiety on him, because he cares for you. —1 Peter 5:7

If you cannot handle your stress, God can. God does a lot more than you know. Just like exercising and eating, prayer, meditation, and giving your stress to God takes practice. There is a reason that it's called

Christian discipline. Discipline takes practice and repetition. You must do things over and over to make them part of how you live your life. Research shows that it takes a new discipline being repeated regularly for about six months to become a habit, and even then we still can slip up.

The good thing is that God is always there to catch us.

THOUGHTS TO PONDER

1. How does stress impact your life?

2. Do you turn to God when you are stressed? Do you feel confident in casting your anxiety upon the Lord and then moving on?

3. How do you think you can improve your stress level?

4. What will you do tomorrow to deal with stress?

Cast all your anxiety on him, because he cares for you. —1 Peter 5:7

DAY 7 Steps taken: _____ Miles journeyed: _____

Exercise chosen: _____

Spiritual thoughts: _____

_____

_____

_____

Feelings: _____

_____

_____

_____

DAY 8 Self-Doubt

BIBLICAL BIG IDEA #8

Truly I tell you, if you have faith and do not doubt, not only will you do what has been done to the fig tree, but even if you say to this mountain, 'Be lifted up and thrown into the sea,' it will be done. —Matthew 21:21

Self-doubt is the evil of not believing in yourself and what you are capable of. Self-doubt can breed sin. We have already determined that you have a reason and meaning for being on the earth. Your body is a tool to get that job done and you have to take care of that tool, just like a car, or a house, or other piece of equipment that is integral to doing the work you are called to in life.

Unfortunately, sometimes self-doubt creeps in. I think I have a self-doubt factory in my brain that spits out messages of "I can't" at regular intervals. First of all, I have the desire to be independent. I like to *think* that I am being self-sacrificing when I won't bother God with the trivial travails of completing my task at hand. I think, surely, God has more important things to worry about than my concerns that I am not being a good mom, I am not handling my colleagues well, I am not finding the time for my ministry, that despite everything that I think and feel, maybe I am not on the right path after all. Doubt can be insidious.

Doubt can also be good, when it fuels the fire of research and questioning, and allows us to delve deeper into the meaning of our relationship with God and how all things come about. I have attained a deeper sense of satisfaction with my spirituality and relationship with God when I have asked the difficult questions and then gone back to the Bible and church teachings. Did that passage really say what I think it said? What does God say about politics, society, government, the needy, or something else? When I doubt, I fail to realize, "With man, this is impossible, but with God, all things are possible" (Matthew 19:26).

Three years ago, my mother was diagnosed with multiple myeloma and it was determined that she would need a bone marrow transplant. She is the primary caregiver for my father, who had a stroke about fifteen years ago. My first job out of nursing school was at a bone marrow transplant unit and, well, let's just say, a lot of people died on my unit. It was an amazing, uplifting, trying, grieving experience working with people who had a terminal illness, but that was with *other* people. I was not ready to face the idea of my *mom* dying. My mom was the rock of my family, and life without her just did not seem possible. I could not comprehend life without Mom.

I was embarrassed that I could not cope with trying to figure out care for my father without my mother. On top of that, being a mom myself, a military wife, and all the other roles we take on, weighed heavy on my plate. I was embarrassed by my emotional response. I like to be strong. I was angry, very angry, that God would bring this on my mother, of whom many people have told me many times, that if there were angels on earth, my mother was one of them.

My mom had enough bad things happen in her life that she did not need to be dealing with cancer on top of it. The fury I felt was palpable. I could not pray and I could not reach out to God; I could not talk to God. I could not even formulate a thought of what I wanted to say about this because my feelings of doubt and fear consumed me. My calling in life and what I thought I should be doing were arrested by the whole situation. I doubted in God, because the first thing that popped into my brain was, "If you are so loving, why would you do this?"

Being a Christian, and having had a relationship with God for some time, I knew that something was very wrong. I knew I needed help. I knew when I couldn't pray on my own and when I couldn't form the very words of petition in my heart that something needed to be done. So I went to see a priest for guidance.

As I met with the priest, it took a long time for me, in my mind, to express my feelings. It was obvious that a parent with cancer, undergoing a bone marrow transplant, is reason enough for concern. I had a multitude of other stressors going on that included a recent move, starting my son in a new school, a search for a new church, work, my dad's health, and unpacking. You name it, I felt like it was on my shoulders. But the root cause of this distress was that I could not imagine my life without my mother and I could not come to terms with this possibility. I could not understand why God would do this to me.

Through my discussion with my priest, I came to realize that my problem came down to doubt. I finally verbalized that if I prayed to God to heal my mother and it did not happen and that she died, I could not understand how I could reconcile God's will with my own will.

At that point in time, I could not see the promise or redemption for myself if my mother was to die. I could not believe that "God's will be done" would be for my mother to die. The anguish that I could not reach out to God in this time was intense. How could I pray in the depths of my soul that I did not think God would save my mother? How could I admit that I wasn't sure God could do it? And if my mother died, would I stop believing in God? (The answer was no, I would still believe in God, I would just be really, really angry for awhile.) I could not let go of my will. I wanted to bend God to my will.

"Abba, Father, for you all things are possible; remove this cup from me; yet, not what I want, but what you want." —Mark 14:36

I could not say this. My doubt was eating me up. It was a sin because not only did it put a barrier between me and God, it effectively put on hold what I was being called to do with my life. Then, something miraculous began to happen.

For where two or three are gathered in my name, I am there among them.
—Matthew 18:20

God was with my priest and me that day and heard my plea. While I felt I could not make myself pray to God about my pain and anger, I was able to verbalize my fears to my priest. Once the words and emotion left me, God still heard and removed my doubts and fears from me. I came to peace that my mother may die. I came to realize that this was not God's will, but rather the nature of the world we live. Whatever may happen, God's will is for God to be with my family and me. I knew then that God would also give me the strength to get through the decisions that would need to be made if she should die regarding how to take care of my dad. I knew, should the worst happen, that through it all, God would wrap my mother in his loving care and she would not be alone.

When I could finally talk to God, "the peace of God which passes all understanding" was amazing. I thank God (and my priest) for finding the time to help me through my doubt. God *does* have the time to deal with it all. My sin is always deciding for God what can and cannot be done and what God may or may not have time for. If I believe that God is omniscient and omnipresent, then I really have no business deciding what God can and cannot do.

So when you have doubt about the hill you may need to climb on your journey or the steps you need to take to finish your goal or the curve in the road you cannot see, keep walking. Keep talking while you walk, knowing that God is there with you and always listening. *Thanks be to God.*

THOUGHTS TO PONDER

1. What are some of your doubts?

2. Have you come to terms with your doubt? Do you have someone you can reach out to, to discuss your doubt and overcome it?

3. How does Jesus' comment "You of little faith, why did you doubt?" (Matthew 14:31) make you feel? Do you doubt?

Immediately he made the disciples get into the boat and go on ahead to the other side, while he dismissed the crowds. And after he had dismissed the crowds, he went up the mountain by himself to pray. When evening came, he was there alone, but by this time the boat, battered by the waves, was far from the land, for the wind was against them. And early in the morning he came walking toward them on the sea. But when the disciples saw him walking on the sea, they were terrified, saying, "It is a ghost!" And they cried out in fear. But immediately Jesus spoke to them and said, "Take heart, it is I; do not be afraid."

Peter answered him, "Lord, if it is you, command me to come to you on the water." He said, "Come." So Peter got out of the boat, started walking on the water, and came toward Jesus. But when he noticed the strong wind he became frightened, and beginning to sink, he cried out, "Lord, save me!" Jesus immediately reached out his hand and caught him, saying to him, "You of little faith, why did you doubt?" —Matthew 14:22–31

DAY 8 Steps taken: _____ Miles journeyed: _____

Exercise chosen: _____

Spiritual thoughts: _____

_____

_____

_____

Feelings: _____

_____

_____

_____

Why We Exercise

BIBLICAL BIG IDEA # 9

For they have no pain; their bodies are sound and sleek.
—Psalm 73:4

In this day and age we have to exercise. Most of us no longer live in a world where our work is exercise and our bodies move as a part of our daily activities of living. Technology has made our lives infinitely easier, yet that much more complex, because now we must work and plan to exercise. Our bodies were designed to move. I know I say this a lot, but really, it's hard for people to understand why their bodies have such a difficult time with weight and exercise when their parents' bodies did not—society has changed drastically.

God gave humans the ability move over all the earth; he did not intend for us to sit in front of the TV. Today, humans spend an average of 8.5 hours in front of screens of some sort (TV, movie, computer, PDA) per day, and this does not lend itself to an active lifestyle. While these activities are enjoyable and allow us to sit and relax away from the chaos of work and school, they do nothing for our bodies. Our environments have evolved, but unfortunately, our bodies are not much different from those of our biblical brothers and sisters. Our bodies expect to till the earth, ride horses or camels, clean on our hands and knees, produce products by hand, and be physically active.

This lack of physical activity has led to a plethora of health problems. It seems that every day scientists identify one more reason we should move. And every day the list of problems that are associated with lack of physical activity are also the same things that can affect our calling in the world. Consider this partial list of impacts of the body that can be improved with physical exercise:

- Obesity
- Tobacco use
- Addiction
- Depression
- Stroke
- Cancer
- Seasonal Affective Disorder
- Premenstrual and menopausal symptoms

- Cardiovascular disease
- Pain control
- Respiratory ailments
- And many more. . .
- Mobility issues

We are just touching the tip of the iceberg on how much we really need to move. I remember returning to work following the birth of my son. I was trying to shed my baby weight and it was proving to be a stubborn task. I telecommute and spend much of my time in front of a computer, either writing for work, writing for Christ Walk, or just connecting with friends and family via the Internet. The older I got, the harder it became to maintain my weight and physical fitness level. I was frustrated. My diet had not changed radically. I have always enjoyed eating healthy and I have always been active. I was completely stumped as to the cause.

I decided to strap a pedometer back on and, lo and behold, I was walking much fewer than 10,000 steps per day. I was simply less active than I had been in the past. This was a wake-up call, since I often feel more active than I really am. Mental work—writing, creating, and training that I do daily—can take a lot of mental energy that can leave me feeling utterly drained at the end of the day. Surely, this equates to running miles! But no, it does not! I had to figure out how to build exercise and movement back into my day in addition to working and taking care of the family.

It honestly is a daily task. Some days I do a better job of fitting the exercise in than other days, and that is okay. Sometimes I get up and expect to exercise and my body is screaming at me for rest. Sometimes we need to listen to our bodies to rest. But overall, we must work extra exercise into our lives. It really does take planning, purpose, and discipline. Just like learning to read the Bible and pray as a Christian discipline, we must now make exercise and eating right a part of that same discipline. If we do not, it will take a toll on our bodies and we will be unable to do those things we were called to do.

If we are not fit, it makes it difficult to keep up with our children. If we are not fit, it makes it difficult to teach our children healthy habits as they grow and develop. If we are not fit, it is difficult to go out there and volunteer and give our time to those in need. If we are not fit, it is difficult to go on missionary journeys. If we are not fit, it is difficult to deal with the stress of our work. If we are not fit, it often becomes hard to pray and develop spiritually, because we are consumed with our bodies not working as we know they should. As we age, if we are not fit, the risk of chronic illness increases dramatically. If we are not fit, the dreams we have for our retirement are replaced by nursing illness.

There are very few people who do not know that they need to exercise more. Rather, the difficulty lies in figuring *how* to incorporate the proper eating and exercise into our lives, because we are bombarded with information on what we should and should not be doing. I do not know about you, but that can send me into a tailspin!

What we need to do is stop, think, and pray about what we CAN do. Because we are not perfect, there isn't anyone in the world who cannot benefit from making lifestyle changes for a healthier self. We ALL have things to work on. It is a lot easier to make those changes one small step at a time. If you decided today to run an Ironman Triathlon and you have never done one before, you might be biting off more than you can chew. However, if you say, this week, I am going to walk 2,000 more steps each day than I did last week and continue doing that, then you will get where you need to be. Our health goals must be set, then updated and revamped as we are able to do more and we are able to go further. It is a continuous journey.

The giving and doing of a Christ-centered life is a lifelong endeavor that will evolve and change. God never intended for us to give our tithe to the church and be done for the day. He never intended for us to do one missionary trip and be good for life. God never intended for us to take up healthy eating and exercising behaviors to then give them up to sloth and gluttony. There will always be one more thing for us to do on this journey, because it's not about us. I have found the greatest satisfaction in my life when I am doing something for others. You would think that was all the encouragement that I would need to continue those behaviors. Unfortunately, I am human, and subject to the human condition that causes me to think of the self and not put God first. Then I get sidetracked on what is right. However, when we stop and put God first, everything else will fall in line.

Let's face it: Exercise is good for you. When you make it a routine and discipline, it feels really good. Keep in mind that it takes repeating a discipline consistently for about six months for it to become a habit. And when it is a habit, then you will know those days when you do not get your exercise. Those are the days when you miss your exercise. This habit of exercise will come, and it will be good for you. You will enjoy it, if you just stick with it. The journey does not end here.

THOUGHTS TO PONDER

1. How do you feel about exercise and a healthy, Christ-centered life?

2. What are small changes you can make today towards the goal you seek?

When you walk, your step will not be hampered; and if you run, you will not stumble. —Proverbs 4:12

DAY 9   Steps taken: _____   Miles journeyed: _____

Exercise chosen: _____

Spiritual thoughts: _____

_____

_____

_____

Feelings: _____

_____

_____

_____

DAY 10 Portion Distortion— Gluttony

BIBLICAL BIG IDEA #10

Therefore I tell you, do not worry about your life, what you will eat or what you will drink, or about your body, what you will wear. Is not life more than food, and the body more than clothing? —Matthew 6:25

I have really struggled about calling this chapter "Gluttony," but then decided to add the concept of "portion distortion" to try to describe this a bit better. The bottom line is that in America, and in more and more developed nations, we suffer from gluttony. Food is bountiful, with great variety and easy access. We do not know what it is like to be hungry and the hunger we do feel on any diet is not the true hunger of those without. Our taste buds are overwhelmed with possibilities. The demand for greater variety has resulted in farming techniques that degrade the nutrition of the foods of the earth. This same demand has bred a revolution of nutritional engineering as people vainly search for the perfect diet food as they try to lose weight from food that is no longer satisfying. As a result, they eat more fake food in a desire to find that satisfaction that these foods no longer provide. Along with the desire to satiate on empty foods, we ingest a great deal of manufactured products that are not necessary for a healthy body. Many times, we are even unaware of what we are putting into our bodies. Even "healthy" foods have ingredient lists with unpronounceable names and additives of which we may be unaware.

God gave us everything we need to be healthy on the earth. That is not to say that the advent of modern medicines and treatments cannot be complementary to natural healing. On the contrary, medicine has made many contributions to health, healing, and disease management that should be a part of a healthy lifestyle. On the other hand, we have also gotten so spoiled by modern medicine that we fail to let our bodies adapt to the environment. We have become so accustomed to quick and easy drugs that we do not give our bodies a chance to try to learn to respond to illness and fight it on its own. We often do not look at our surrounding environment and the food we put into our bodies as some of the possible culprits for the illnesses or diseases we may be fighting. Some of the illnesses we face today are simply because we did not think of the consequences of our choices. We pop pills with abandon, looking for quick fixes for illnesses that might resolve on their own, or may improve with lifestyle changes. The first step to managing your health is to look at the food you put in your body.

I love food. I love REAL food, food that I know what it is and where it came from. If I am lucky, which I am not always, I have talked to the farmer and participated in local food production (such as community supported agriculture programs—CSAs—or farmers' markets). Utilizing CSAs or farmers' markets, I know what has happened to my food, what has been put on it, and how far it has traveled to get to my table. I do not have the luxury, or the talent, to grow my own food, so it is important to me to research and find the best food for my family and myself. I know that when my family eats the best food possible for us, we are happier and healthier and better able to adapt. Real food can be good food. That doesn't mean eating only raw (although that works for some people) and doesn't necessarily mean eating mostly protein (although that works from some people) and I do not think that you have to cut out all dairy or wheat (although that works for some people) unless that is what works for you. The core of many of these diets is that they are getting back to real food.

The problem with processed food is that it goes through so many changes that it is not real food once it gets to you. Many ingredients are stripped from the recipes and then added back again as additives later in the process. Depending on the food and the necessity of a long shelf life, many types of fillers and preservatives are included as well.

These foods are engineered to be addictive. Food scientists work on designing the perfect snack food to satisfy either sweet or salty or bitter taste and wrap it in textures that are irresistible. Over time, these foods build up a "need" in our systems in order to eat more and feel satisfied. This is no different than an addictive drug. These are the same foods that fill our bodies with empty calories and empty satisfaction. Soon we think these foods make us feel better and therefore can be the heal-all for mental concerns, stress, irritability, fatigue, and feeling morose. Then we rely on these foods instead of our relationship with God, and our bodies get sick. Just as our bodies were designed to move, our bodies were designed to eat the fruits, grains, fish, fowl, and meat of the earth. Genesis 1:28–30 is all about the abundance of good things in the world that the Lord has given us for sustenance. We need to get back to real food.

Not only has the quality of food changed, but also our approach to eating has changed. We are seated (hopefully), given a plate of food, and are expected to clear the food in order to prevent waste. Plates, bowls, and cups are larger than in previous years. We place our expectation of satiety on portion size rather than on what our bodies tell us we need. The body will tell you when you need more food. This time period varies from person to person. Some individuals need three large meals and others need six small meals. Others can go on one or two meals a day and others could graze randomly throughout their waking hours. The important thing is learning to listen to your body.

When it comes to weight loss, most of the diets in the world are based on a calorie deficit. Some of these weight-loss diets may trick you into thinking you are getting more than you are, but there are two rules of thumb with weight loss and eating:

1. If it sounds too good to be true, it probably is.

2. It takes a deficit of about 3,500 calories to burn a pound of fat.

Over the course of a week, your calorie intake needs to be 500 calories less than your calorie output per day in order to burn one pound. In addition you will have to eat the right kind of food to stimulate this weight loss. The RIGHT kind of foods, in the RIGHT amount for your activity level, are the keys to a healthy diet.

Many people do not realize how much they eat. That is why if you are choosing to include weight loss as a part of your Christ Walk you need to write down everything that you put in your mouth and track those calories. There are many applications for smart phones and computers that can help you do this for free. You do not need to spend a lot of money to do this. You do need to take some time to find out how much fuel your body needs, how it feels when it is really hungry, and how much you actually do put into your body to fuel it.

We need to understand that so much diet food available is processed carbs. These do not help you lose weight. God did not hang meal replacement bars in the Garden of Eden. There are recent studies to suggest that diets high in carbohydrates, especially processed carbohydrates, make it very difficult to lose weight. You may have the appropriate caloric deficit to lose weight, but if you are filling your diet with nothing but carbs, your body is not getting a variety of nutrients to work efficiently at fat burning. This is why I am a fan of a diet that is real: real fruits and vegetables, real meat, and minimally processed grains in small portions.

During Lent some religious traditions have two major fast days: Ash Wednesday and Good Friday. These are fast days to remember the forty days and nights that Jesus fasted in the desert, avoiding temptation, and preparing his body for what he would be called to do in the coming days. Jesus knew that the body needed to fast in order to prepare for the different things he was being called to do in his life. We also need to look at food and exercise as preparation for what our bodies are called to do. If you are able to complete a one-day fast, it is a wonderful experience. It can let the bowel rest, it can clear the body of toxins, and it can let you reacquaint your body with what hunger really feels like. When I fast, I usually do a clear liquid/juice fast that pumps my body up with antioxidants, is easy to digest, and gives me just enough fuel to get through my day. Unlike times past, there are very few of us who stop our jobs and lives to spend the day solely in contemplative prayer in order to truly fast and rest. Fasting allows you to leave your worries about food behind and focus on your spiritual hunger and prayers. Fasting can be a really good experience for you and your body to get reacquainted with the signals it sends. However, before fasting, you should discuss this with your health-care provider to ensure your body is able to fast safely.

I have mentioned that I love food. Does this mean that I have never eaten junk food? On the contrary, I have a special weakness for pizza and love to eat a dinner that ends with a nice chocolaty dessert. Does this mean that I think that chocolate, ice cream, pizza, drinks, etc., are bad? No, I don't. I think that what we need to do when we choose our indulgence foods is:

1. Remember that indulgences are treats. Somewhere around college, I started thinking that every day was a treat day and that every evening was a dessert evening. Make these indulgences a special occasion and savor (the smell, the taste, the texture, the look, the sound) every moment of it.

2. Choose your indulgences wisely. I am far more satisfied with one really good piece of dark chocolate than I am with an entire bar of random milk chocolate.

3. Practice moderation. If you sit in front of the TV with a bag of potato chips and mindlessly eat through the bag with no awareness of what you are doing, you are not doing anything good for your body. You will also overeat.

4. Make sure your indulgences are real food: real cheese, real chocolate, real potatoes, etc. You will be satisfied with a smaller portion of a real food version of your indulgence than a processed version.

Unfortunately, many of us are not aware of what our weaknesses are and are unable to practice moderation. Until you have gotten your weaknesses under control and you are comfortable practicing moderation, I would advise against eating your trigger foods. These foods can be just as bad as any other addiction like drugs, tobacco, or alcohol if they are controlling you, instead of you controlling them.

THOUGHTS TO PONDER

1. How do you feel about food?

2. Do you have trigger foods? Cravings?

3. What can you do to help control those cravings and trigger foods? What can you do to practice moderation?

4. How do you feel about fasting? Can you make it a spiritual experience?

5. Can you make changes in your life that are a gift to God?

But when you fast, put oil on your head and wash your face, so that your fasting may be seen not by others but by your Father who is in secret; and your Father who sees in secret will reward you. —Matthew 6:17–19

DAY 10   Steps taken: _____   Miles journeyed: _____

Exercise chosen: _____

Spiritual thoughts: _____

_____

_____

_____

Feelings: _____

_____

_____

_____

DAY 11 Mental Health— My Dad's Story

BIBLICAL BIG IDEA #11
Anxiety weighs down the human heart. —Proverbs 12:25

Five percent of the American population deals with some type of serious mental disorder. Mental illness is a silent and deadly disease that affects the person and their friends, family, and colleagues. Mental illness can manifest itself through physical symptoms as well as personality changes and erratic behavior. Sometime mental illness can be very insidious. Sometimes it can present itself as simple withdrawal from those around you, and can quickly escalate into increasing abnormal behavior.

I feel the need to speak frankly about mental illness, as my father has struggled with mental illness for the last twenty to twenty-five years. It is difficult to pinpoint when it first started, but my father was in a training accident in the Navy and lost consciousness. In today's military, my father would have been diagnosed with a traumatic brain injury, but back then, the diagnosis was not as common. Unbeknownst to the doctors, my father was having complex partial seizures in the area of his brain that controlled his personality. Initially, the only symptom my dad had was that he would rub his first finger against his thumb. In fact, over the years, he had rubbed this area raw and we honestly just thought it was a nervous twitch. I am sure that my father suffered from mild depression before his accident, but the accident triggered this depression to spiral out of control. Back then, the stigma of anyone admitting depression, let alone a military officer and chaplain, would have been a career-ending move. Slowly, my father's depression became more pronounced, and he began having personality changes and violent mood swings that baffled and confused us. He started smoking again after many years of abstinence. He would say odd things and act very paranoid about situations. He was unable to do the work he was called to do as a priest and his work life deteriorated. This was not the man I remembered when growing up.

My memory of my father is one who took the time to put together toys on Christmas morning and roughhouse on the den floor in the evening. He worked hard, but we also had fun. I treasure that memory of my dad on Christmas morning, because this is how I choose to remember him. While he was always a deep thinker and sensitive to the ills of the world, the man that came out during his mental illness was not the man I remember as my father. It took the doctors over five years to realize that these manifestations were from seizures rather than manic-depressive episodes. And it took several more years to finally make his depression manageable with the right drugs for the right diagnosis. My mother was a rock during this time. She laughs it off and says she wasn't, but she was. She was a rock because she prayed, and she was a rock because she did not have much choice in the matter.

We had, and have, a lot of opportunities with my dad to "what if." I often dream of what life might have been like had he not suffered from his illness. I often wonder if things would have been different had there not been a stigma associated with mental illness, but I also look back on those years and know we did the best we could with the information we had. We knew something was wrong with my dad. We knew the initial treatment and diagnosis plan was not working and, unfortunately, it took my dad getting to the point of being suicidal before he got the help he needed.

Did my father ever return to the man I remember on Christmas mornings? No, he did not, but with prayer and realization that mental disorders are an illness, I could remove my anger and blame from my dad and place it squarely at the feet of the depression. It is very difficult for families of patients with mental illness to separate the illness from the person they know and love, because these illnesses change those personalities that they first fell in love with and know. Mental illness affects more than just the individual.

Mental illness also does not have to be as severe as my father's. It could be worse, or it could be extremely mild. Anxiety that cannot be controlled, unnecessary worrying, blue moods that do not resolve themselves, fear of being around others, fear of work, overeating, over drinking, and anger are all potential signs that something is not ticking quite right in your brain.

Anxiety weighs down the human heart. —Proverbs 12:25

All these symptoms, if they are not addressed, can spiral out of control. Perhaps if we had addressed my dad's milder symptoms early on, the results from his accident would not have been so severe.

Worrying about "what-ifs" weighs a person down. Anxiety weighs the body down. Mental illness causes you to lose your vitality and luster, as well as the ability to cope and interact. I also believe that mental illness can make it extremely difficult to pray, since it separates you from everything. It is also difficult to pray and understand what you are praying for when you often do not even know what started the problem to begin with. Illness in the heart can fester for many years before presenting as a really serious condition.

Health is of the mind, body, and spirit. If you are concerned about your mental health, I urge you to talk to someone to find out what can be done. There is no shame in seeking help. If your heart was not ticking right, you would go to a cardiologist; if your brain is not ticking right then you should go see a behavioral health specialist. Sometimes just talking about what weighs on the mind is the best way to get it out of your system. Remember when my mom's illness was weighing so heavy on my heart that I could not function? Well, just talking about it got me over that hump. I did not need medications or therapy, I just needed to get it out of my system by talking. This also may be what you need. Or maybe you need something more intensive. This is okay. It is worth it for your job, your family, and your friends to take care of your mental health.

While my dad will never return to the same man that I remember growing up with, he has found a sense of balance that works for him and my mother after many years of drug trials and therapy. He continued to smoke initially and then sixteen years ago he had a stroke. Ironically, the stroke caused him to forget about smoking. He has no recollection of the habit now and, sometimes, I see glimpses of the man I remembered growing up.

The stroke caused full paralysis of his right side and he has little speech. Through therapy, he is able to move around with a leg brace and use his left arm to feed and clothe himself. He is unable to play with his grandkids, to throw a ball, or run around with them. He cannot teach them to fish or bike or use tools. He cannot read them stories. However, although he is unable to communicate with speech, he finds ways to continue to share himself with those around him. He still has a twinkle in his eye.

If I dwell on what could have been, had he not had this mental illness, I miss out on the opportunity to create a relationship and memories with my dad as he is now. I cannot change the past; I can only work with what I have now to make memories for the future. I could hate my father for what we went through, but that does little for *my* mind, body, or spiritual health and my anger will change nothing. I love my dad. He still makes me smile and while I wish more than anything he could be the granddad to my kids that I always wanted, it is okay that he is not. He is still sharing his light in the world.

And everyone in this world with a mental illness has a light to share in this world.

Thanks be to God.

THOUGHTS TO PONDER

1. Are you anxious, worried, and fearful? Does it control your life?

2. Do you think you need to talk to someone about it? Does your family think you should talk to someone about it?

3. What would God tell you to do?

4. Do you think you are worthy of this love? What can you do to bask in the Lord's love forever?

O give thanks to the God of gods, for his steadfast love endures forever.
—Psalm 136:2

DAY 11 Steps taken: _____ Miles journeyed: _____

Exercise chosen: _____

Spiritual thoughts: _____

_____

_____

_____

Feelings: _____

_____

_____

_____

12 Temptations

BIBLICAL BIG IDEA #12:

Stay awake and pray so that you may not come into the time of trial; the spirit indeed is willing, but the flesh is weak.
—Matthew 26:41

The world is full of temptations. These temptations can lead us to sin. God gave us freedom of thought and movement to make choices. We often want to go back and blame God for mistakes that we make because of poor choices, but we cannot have it both ways. We cannot ask God to fix things here and there, but then turn around and demand the freedom to make our own choices. Just as we do with our children, God loves us greatly. God has given us the guidebook on how to live our lives and lets us go make those mistakes and choices that this freedom allows us.

Everywhere we turn there are temptations that conflict with a healthy life. Temptations are things we know we should be doing, but choose to do another. Sin is when we fail to communicate with God throughout it all. Sin is when we knowingly make a choice that we should not make that drives us further from God.

When it comes to a healthy life, temptations are difficult. If I have set the path of healthy eating, then ice cream, cake, cookies, and chips become temptations. These things are not necessarily bad if enjoyed in small portions, but I have the tendency to look at every day as a celebration of something and will happily enjoy these treats every day if I allow myself. When I eat these things, I have filled myself with food that, while enjoyable, takes up room from the fruits, vegetables, and grains of the earth that power my body and keep it healthy. A steady diet of junk food is not healthy; it does not give me the nutrients and antioxidants my body needs to fight disease and illness. The more fake food you put in your system, the less able it is to handle the stress of life.

When I look at my exercise habits, my temptations are the desire to put off my exercise in lieu of time on the couch with a book or a movie. Quiet times are so few and far between that my temptation is to put off my exercise. The only person I cheat is me because my exercise is good for me and keeps me strong for the things I am called to do in life.

The negligence of putting my prayer discipline second in my life is my most difficult temptation. Life gets in the way of my spiritual discipline all the time. I much prefer to have an ongoing conversation with God in my head during the day than to purposefully sit down in prayer and worship. I get too busy. I get too distracted. But just like any other relationship, when I do not nurture my relationship in God, it suffers due to my temptations. Initially, the only person that suffers from your temptations is you. Your physical, mental, and spiritual health will deteriorate from your temptations. Some temptations spiral out of control and begin to take over your life. Some temptations start to affect those around you (think about the "three most important things" exercise).

What are temptations? Temptations are those things that keep you from doing what you should. The thing itself is not necessarily evil, but what we do with the thing can breed temptation and evil. If that temptation comes in the way of what we *should* be doing, then it is a sin that needs to be addressed. You will need to work on your actions through prayer to overcome that temptation. *Everyone* has temptations. No matter how godly your life or how much grace you experience, at some point you will be faced with temptations.

One of the hardest things to do is to learn to walk away from temptations. Say a prayer; look at the temptation, and say, "You will not rule my life." I will do what is good for me first. If your temptation is something that is dangerous for you or your family and you cannot control it, you need to use the power of the Holy Spirit to walk away from it forever. Sometimes, you will need to leverage experienced professionals to help you.

"Things" are not sinful; what we do with those things is what causes sin. Having a glass of wine is not sinful; however, if I drink two bottles of wine in a night and am unable to take care of my children and do my job, that thing has become my temptation and causes me to sin. Some people believe that things of high temptation should be banned so as not to cause people to sin. That is not my personal theology. I am responsible for my actions and I must learn to take control and responsibility for them. Can you truly ask God's forgiveness if you do not understand why you have sinned and what has caused you to sin?

Temptations come in all different shapes and sizes; some temptations are at the crossroads of what society deems acceptable and what is God's law. Consider these temptations:

• Food	• Promiscuity	• Money
• Alcohol	• The quick fix	• Envy
• Drugs	• Vanity	• Speed

- Laziness
- Fad diets
- Spitefulness

- Greed
- Pills
- And many more.

- Anger
- Work

None of these things in excess are good for mind, body, and spiritual health. All of these things in excess are damaging to the three most important things in your life. Tap into your spiritual toolbox of prayer, physical exercise, church, friends, and support groups in order to address your temptations. It is okay to have temptations, we all do, we are all human; the problem is when these temptations take over our lives and keep us from what we are called to do. Every person on earth has a calling; we all have a purpose for being here.

Everyone is going to have different sins and temptations they need to address as a part of a healthy life. Temptations become less tempting when we acknowledge them and develop strategies that teach us how to deal with them. When we have learned those strategies, we have made ourselves that much stronger. If we have used our relationship with God to help deal with those temptations, then we have drawn that much closer to God.

But for God all things are possible. —Matthew 19:26

Through God we can overcome anything.

Later we will talk about strategies for dealing with temptations and keeping a healthy life a priority of mind, body, and spiritual balance. I KNOW you can do this. I know that God has given us the tools and he has given us amazing forgiveness for when we slip up. It's the getting up and moving on again that is success.

THOUGHTS TO PONDER

1. What are your temptations?

2. Do they rule your life? Do you have a coping strategy for overcoming temptation? What is it?

3. What do you think of your temptation in relationship to sin and the three most important things in your life?

No testing has overtaken you that is not common to everyone. God is faithful, and he will not let you be tested beyond your strength, but with the testing he will also provide the way out so that you may be able to endure it.
—1 Corinthians 10:13

DAY 12 Steps taken: _____ Miles journeyed: _____

Exercise chosen: _____

Spiritual thoughts: _____

_____

_____

_____

_____

Feelings: _____

_____

_____

_____

_____

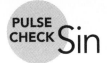

PULSE CHECK Sin

There are a number of things that *can* be a sin. "Things" do not *make* us sin. We sin because we are human and we sin through the choices we make. We sin when we pit our will against God's will and what we want to do against what we should do. This leads us to separate ourselves from God due to shame, doubt, guilt, fear, embarrassment, and ignorance. This separation from God is the greatest sin of all. When we stop talking to God and forget to work through fears and doubts with God, then we sin. When we believe that we are capable of dealing with problems and frustrations on our own without God, we sin.

Sin is an unfortunate part of human nature. When God gave us freedom to choose, he allowed us the choice between a godly life and our own selfish pursuits. Righteous men and women put God first in *all* the decisions of their lives. It isn't that they don't have temptations or sin; righteous men and women have woven their relationship with God into dealing with sin and temptation. The sinful individual does not talk to God or consider God in the context of the choices he or she may make.

Because we are not divine, we are flawed. Sin is a part of human nature. However, God's grace gives us the strength to move past sin. Only through God's redeeming grace do we have the opportunity for forgiveness and love and starting over each time with God. God can lift us above any sin. God is infinitely forgiving. He will forgive as many times as it takes because the crucifixion of Christ paid any debt we may incur for our sins. Forgiveness is free to all who choose the gift of God's love. And forgiveness happens over and over because we sin over and over. To sin or not to sin is the choice we made when we decided that abiding in the Garden of Eden was not enough. And God loves us enough to make those choices and still be there with us through it all. Sin is a part of the human condition.

PART THREE

JUDGMENT

13 Slipping Up

BIBLICAL BIG IDEA #13:

Though we stumble, we shall not fall headlong, for the Lord holds us by the hand. —Psalm 37:24

I find resolutions the easiest to keep during Lent. I tend to think along the lines of, "By golly, if Jesus could fast for forty days and forty nights, then surely I can stick with my simple fasting promise as well." I find it very appropriate that it is Lent as I write this section and I have given up caffeine, sugar, and alcohol as part of my fasting regimen to clear my body and prepare it for the work to come. Winter leaves the body feeling slow and sluggish and not yet awake. I find my Lenten fast a wonderful opportunity to wake it up and feel healthy once again. It is a shame that I feel the need to do this every year. I would like to think that I do a good job of keeping the temple healthy throughout the year, but the truth is, every year I need to get back to the basics. I am humbled every Lent that God's strength holds me up and makes me strong.

Lent is the period during the church year when we remember when Jesus went into the mountains for forty days and nights to be tempted by Satan. During Lent, some Christians practice "giving up" poor behaviors and habits or "taking up" good practices and habits to lead a more Christ-like life during these forty days. This discipline of giving up or taking on prepares us for the gift of Christ's crucifixion. Lent is a perfect time to spiritually consider how you can devote yourself more to God.

As humans, we are far from perfect. You are not perfect and you will never be perfect except by the grace of God. Our bodies are not perfect. We will not approach health perfectly. We will make mistakes and bad decisions. Some of the decisions we make we know are bad choices. Other decisions we make ignorant of the impact of those choices. We are called to do the best we can with the tools we have. We will be faced with temptation and there will be days when we slip up. We will be faced with temptation, but, by the Grace of God, we will persevere towards healthier choices. We can strive towards perfection, but I do not believe that perfection happens here on earth.

This is okay, because by the grace of our Lord Jesus Christ, we are forgiven for our sins and our slip-ups. However, I believe that as a Christian my duty after slipping up is to pray for forgiveness and then get back up on my feet to do what is right. If I have simply prayed for forgiveness and continued with my sin, am I truly repentant in my heart? If I remain guilty for my slip-up or sin, have I truly let God into my heart to cleanse me of my sin and move on? Have I accepted the forgiveness of God if I continue to dwell and have anxiety over my sin? If my sin is as far as the east is from the west once God has forgiven me (Psalm 103:12), then I, too, need to put my sin aside, know that I am worthy of God's forgiveness, and move on. No matter what you have done, you are worthy of forgiveness. Through forgiveness we are open to acts of repentance, which lead to redemption.

We all have transgressions in our life (remember no one is perfect) and we will have more transgressions, no matter how righteous a life we try to live. Either by omission, action, or word we will fail to do unto others as we should. My transgressions as a human are many. My prayers for forgiveness are many. I like to think that since we have a kind and loving God, as long as I continue to strive towards a Christian life (even when I make mistakes), God will understand. And then the next time I am faced with the same sin, hopefully I will not slip up (although that has been known to happen as well!).

While doing Christ Walk, and when we try to make changes in our lives (think about what you wrote down that you want most to change about yourself), we will slip up. As I have mentioned previously, it often takes disciplined repetition of a habit for around six months for it to become a lifelong habit. Even when we have established a new habit for six months we can still regress. Sometimes we do not know we are slipping up along the way of a healthy life. I remember after the birth of my second child that I was heavy and out of shape and I could not for the life of me figure out what happened. I was busy chasing two kids, nursing, and working. I still walked and exercised. I did not *think* my diet was all that bad, and yet I could not get back into shape. It took me several years to figure out how to get back on track. This from the woman who has worked in the health care field for many years! I used to teach people how to have a healthy life and I was embarrassed at how out of shape I had let my body become. I was too tired to have time for my kids. I think I took for granted my previous ability to quit eating dessert or some other minor change to my life to lose weight. I did not have to count calories; I just needed to be sensible about my eating. Usually, I returned to my normal weight, but this time I struggled. Well, life and bodies change. Now, if

I have to lose weight and get back into shape, I have to track it, write it down, and be mindful of it. These are the things that help keep me from slipping up.

Another difficult thing about starting a lifestyle change is that the starting up can be uncomfortable. When I begin my Lenten fast of cleansing alcohol, caffeine, and sugar from my system, I usually feel worse before I feel better. Building the temple is not an overnight event. Jesus may have been able to tear down a temple and rebuild it in three days; however we humans take a little bit longer to make changes to our personal bodies. When we attempt to make change, there is often a lot of initial discomfort that can cause us to slip up and give up. However, if we stick with it and allow our bodies to adjust, eventually we feel the terrific benefits of building a stronger body. When I started running, I hurt. It took a long time for it to feel right, and even now it is still hard work. Nothing that is worthwhile in life is easy.

Slipping up for different people can mean different things:

- Chocolate cake
- Ice cream
- Coffee
- Alcohol
- Drugs
- Stress
- Pizza
- Brownies
- Cookies
- Soda
- Bread
- Pasta
- Chips
- Skipping a workout
- Candy
- Anger
- Foul speech
- Unkind words
- Adultery

Slipping up is usually one of our temptations that we have not been able to moderate. When you are slipping up, or feeling imminent failure, please pray. Open your heart and let your angst and worry fall on God's shoulders so that you can be lifted up and carried through the next hump of your journey. The journey NEVER stops. I do not believe that life here on earth is the end. I think there will be another journey around the bend and many different journeys in a lifetime and in God's time.

So when you slip up, ask forgiveness, stand yourself up, dust yourself off, and start again. You are worth it. God does forgive you and the road does not end here. Be at peace.

THOUGHTS TO PONDER

1. Have you slipped up? Has it kept you from getting back up and going again?

2. Do you feel guilt about slipping up? Do you have difficulty in accepting God's forgiveness for your sins?

3. If so, what can you do about it?

Happy are those whose transgression is forgiven, whose sin is covered.
—Psalm 32:1

DAY 13 Steps taken: _____ Miles journeyed: _____

Exercise chosen: _____

Spiritual thoughts: _____

_____

_____

_____

Feelings: _____

_____

_____

_____

14 Risk Factors

BIBLICAL BIG IDEA #14:

Those who are well have no need of a physician, but those who are sick. —Luke 5:31

Not all health problems are related to what we do to ourselves. Every person comes with a set of risk factors in their genetic makeup that make them more likely to be affected by certain diseases and illnesses. I also think there are individuals who, because of their genetic makeup, are *less* likely to be affected by disease and illness. This is just the way we are made. Perhaps it is our parents' mix of genes, or environmental factors, or perhaps sociological, cultural, and economic factors that can impact our health risk. We are all given a bag of flawed cells that we have to make the best of. No one is perfect.

There is risk in walking across a street. Everyone runs a risk of getting hit by a car. However, to offset risk, you can look both ways, use a crosswalk, or avoid crossing the street. This decreases your risk of getting hit by a car.

Health risk is similar. Due to our genes, gender, race, economic situation, and family history, we all have risks. A family history of a problem can increase your risk for certain diseases because it gets passed down on the genetic code that makes you, you. Risk factors impact risk for cancer, heart disease, stroke, diabetes, depression, obesity, asthma, allergies, autoimmune disease, and many other problems. Your genetic code also impacts your ability to be resilient to adverse factors and how you bounce back from adverse events. This code also makes your body more or less likely to be affected by disease and disability depending on how resilient your body may be. In a way, there is a sort of predestination to how we are made up physically and mentally.

However, just as with walking across a street, you can offset health risk factors with choices. This is one of the joys of the freedom that God gave us. The genes we are given do not solely determine our future; our future is also determined by the choices we make. We have the ability to make choices that can lead to a better and healthier life. I believe that through

God, we can make the right choices. I believe God will lift us up and help us to make the right choices so that the temple of our bodies is strong. I believe that we should allow God to be a part of our health. Doctors did not design the body. God designed the body. I want to ensure that God is with me making the decisions about my body, even as I talk to my doctor about the right choices.

If you choose to walk in front of busy traffic while jaywalking, you increase the probability of getting hit by a car. If you have a family history of heart disease and choose not to exercise or eat healthfully, then you increase your probability of a heart attack or other heart disease. We often do not want to walk the healthier road as it takes thinking, preparing, discernment, and will. We need to retrain our bodies to love healthy food. We have set patterns of inactivity and need to reawaken our bodies to being active. By being active and making healthy eating choices, we are taking a first step towards offsetting risk factors. We need to make health choices a priority of our Christian lives.

An additional problem with risk factors is that it puts us in a state of conflict between what we want to do and what we should do. This is life, and every decision we make is a comparison between what we should do and what we want to do. Whichever choice we make, there are consequences, and we need to be prepared to accept the results of the choices we make. If we choose to eat poorly and not exercise, our temple will weaken and fall. We need to be cognizant of those choices and own up to them. If you continue to smoke, knowing the risks of that habit, then that's fine.

However, that choice is yours and you need to know the consequences of your habit on yourself, your health, your family, your job, and your healthcare options. You can still be a good Christian and own up to your choices, and perhaps today is not the day when you want to critically examine those choices and make changes. Perhaps that will be tomorrow, or in a year, or in ten years. The great news is that there is no time limit on God's forgiveness and willingness to help us through those choices.

If we look back historically on the impact of choices, we see that this has been going on since the beginning. God granted Adam and Eve freedom of choice, and they chose to sin. We all have that same choice. The gift of the freedom of choice is that there is always going to be a decision to be made. If God is not at the heart of your decision-making process, then you run the risk of making poor decisions. Sometimes the decisions that you will make with God will conflict with what society says is "right." Stick with your decisions that are made with God and do not worry about what society thinks.

God did not say that our life as Christians would be easy. In fact, God was pretty confident that we would be persecuted and reviled for our relationship with him. God does not ask us to live in communion with secular life, God asks us to live in communion with him, creation, and one another.

With the gift of freedom, the choices of many millennia have played out in our bodies. We cannot know the impact of our decisions today on the world of tomorrow and years to come. For better or worse, we did not know that additives in our food to preserve it and make it abundant might create a slew of allergies and reactions and contribute to poor digestion. For better or worse, we do not know the impact of genetically tweaking our food. For better or worse, we do not know the impact of medical advances. We may see these advances as a godsend, and in later years realize there was a greater impact on the population than we realized. This is why medicine is not God. We do not know but God does. We all must just do the very best we can with the knowledge and skills and abilities that we have and do it to God's glory. No matter what we do, we will all die. If we are in communion with God throughout all these choices and doing the best we can, God will continue to be with us in the end. In the meantime, we need to think and pray and work on our choices and decision-making.

With these decisions and risk factors comes the need to make healthy choices. I like to think the choices that make me healthier bring me that much closer to God. When I am well and making good decisions, then I am moving more in God's love and that is a good thing.

We all have risk factors for diseases. We all have things that will play against us no matter what. We may get ill no matter how healthy our lifestyle. We must just do the best job we can. God is with us through it all. God gave us the gift of freedom to do what we will with our bodies. God also wants us to make the choice to be in relationship with him during times of health, not just during times of illness or low points. A dear friend of mine calls the low points of life a part of "the human condition." Life is the result of the human condition. Bad things happen as the result of the human condition. What makes the human condition worthwhile is the relationship we have with God through all parts of life. God is always seeking a relationship with us and we should always seek one with him.

THOUGHTS TO PONDER

1. What are my risk factors?

2. Does my lifestyle increase or decrease my risk factors? (If you do not know, consider talking to someone who can help you answer this question.)

3. If you are hit with a terrible illness, will you blame God, or will you seek to have a relationship with him in spite of these things happening? How do you feel about the human condition?

The LORD sustains them on their sickbed; in their illness you heal all their infirmities. —Psalm 41:3

DAY 14   Steps taken: _____   Miles journeyed: _____

Exercise chosen: _____

Spiritual thoughts: _____

_____

_____

_____

Feelings: _____

_____

_____

_____

15 Physical Exercise for Health

BIBLICAL BIG IDEA #15:

I pray that all may go well with you and that you may be in good health, just as it is well with your soul. —3 John 1:2

We must exercise for our physical health. No longer do the labors of our days work our muscles and heart and keep our bodies strong; rather, we sit and work our minds. This can lead our bodies to atrophy, illness, and disease. It is well established in scientific literature how important it is that we move our bodies and stay strong and healthy. The human body was designed to move.

We need to exercise. The great thing is that you are making those strides with every step you add in this forty-day journey. We are walking this forty-day journey to add more and more steps to our life in an effort to keep moving a little farther and a little longer. You are making strides to a healthier you and a healthier temple. I could not be more proud. Sticking with a program for two weeks thus far is a huge, momentous step in the right direction. We are one-third of the way through and, hopefully, by the end you will have established a lifestyle change to continue this exercise throughout your life. I hope that you are finding the right balance between prayer, work, physical exercise, and the healthy choices that God is showing you.

But as usual, our own weaknesses may be getting in the way of making those right choices. I hope that you are praying to God each night to give you the strength and fortitude to take on the next step. Taking on physical exercise can be very daunting if you have never done it before. Our own weaknesses can be very destructive; they constantly ring a refrain of "I can't" in the back of our minds. This is where we need to strengthen our minds, or look at ways of modification to take on the next step.

I have never said that anyone taking on this journey must train for a marathon by the end of it (although you could); however, just as a runner does not go out and run 26.2 miles the first time they hit the road, they use a training plan, we are going to develop a plan.

First, choose something you like to do. Whatever exercise you choose, find a training plan to follow. Most individuals who are physically active have chosen an exercise they enjoy. If you do not like walking, then choose your "steps" in another fashion. I believe I have exercise ADD—I very rarely do anything consistently enough to get really good add it, but I switch it up constantly so that I do not get bored. As a result, I am always working to improve the type of exercise I am currently doing. Some days I walk, others I bike, swim, run, lift weights, hike, kayak, or do yoga. I listen to my body and I think of what will excite me today to try, and then I go do that. During that time of exercise, I am usually talking to God about what I do or do not like about what I am doing and how I can become better at it. Sometimes, I let the repetition of the movement quiet my mind, so God can speak to me in his mysterious ways and I can hear the calling in my life. I like the quiet moments in my mind that exercise brings me. I sometimes feel like a cartoon character on my runs when a light bulb goes off in my head and a wonderful, "A-ha!" moment occurs. God has never failed to send me a message when I have opened my mind and released my expectations. Something comes; it may not be what I expected, but I always get a message. This usually happens for me when I am exercising and praying at the same time.

Which leads me to a discussion on expectations: I am the queen of expectations. Your expectation for the end of this journey may have been to go farther than you are able in your exercise. That is an exemplary goal! But sometimes, we need to let go of our expectations and enjoy the journey and enjoy the fact that we are simply moving when we have not moved before. Tomorrow may be the day when you can increase your walk to a jog, or your jog to a run. But it might not be today. As they say, "Rome was not built in a day." Your physical exercise routine is going to have to evolve. Let go of your expectations for your exercise and just enjoy the daily journey.

Physical exercise IS good for your health. It is the number one activity that can reduce the effects of almost any illness or disease. The more you exercise, the better it feels. The more you exercise, the stronger it makes you. The stronger you are, the more work you can do in the world.

Many large corporations are incorporating physical exercise into their benefits packages by including gyms or memberships or flex time for exercise. This is because they have seen that healthier employees are more productive, cost less on their insurance plans and, all in all, bring more to the table than their sedentary counterparts. Our ability to take on physical exercise is a part of God's benefit package to us in the world and the work we do for him. Doing work in the world is a part of the bottom line for God's corporation and we are all employees in that organization. When you accept God's love and forgiveness in your life, you reap the benefit of everlasting life. When you accept the gift of physical exercise and healthy eating, then you reap the benefit of a strong body to do God's work in the world. It is all good.

If you are struggling this week with sticking to your steps, try something new. Switch it up—try a weight lifting class, or yoga, or tai-chi. Center yourself in the exercise and let God flow through you with whatever you are choosing to do today. But unless you are injured, don't stop. Keep working at the journey because it will only be better for you in the end. If you are injured, talk to your healthcare provider about what you can do to get back on the road to health. There are many low-impact options that may work for you, including swimming or water aerobics. Remember that every fifteen minutes of exercise is worth a mile. Don't stop. You are doing great and you will continue to get better as long as you stick with it.

The road to increased physical exercise does not end at the end of these forty days. You will be constantly challenged on how to fit in physical exercise, make healthy eating choices, and make the right decisions for your temple. When God destroyed the temple in Jerusalem, I believe he rebuilt it in each of us with the blood of his forgiveness of our sins. I believe that God's grace alone is the gift of our salvation, but what we do with that gift is just as important. Too often, we put the gift of our salvation and God's love on a pedestal to be admired from afar. This does not resonate for me. I believe that just like physical exercise and healthy eating and healthy spirit, my gift of salvation belongs to others. I am not here for me. Yes, I enjoy the journey, but while I do not believe that I must *work* for my salvation, I believe that it is a poor testament to God's gift, if I do nothing. My father brought me up with the saying, "A faith without works is no faith."

God's peace to you in your exercise this week.

THOUGHTS TO PONDER

1. Am I in a rut with my routine? Am I being self-sabotaging with my exercise?

2. What can I do to switch it up?

3. Am I feeling healthier? If so, what can I do to take it to the next level?

4. Where do I want to go with my goal?

Not that I have already obtained this or have already reached the goal; but I press on to make it my own, because Christ Jesus has made me his own. Beloved, I do not consider that I have made it my own; but this one thing I do: forgetting what lies behind and straining forward to what lies ahead.
—Philippians 3:12–13

DAY 15   Steps taken: _____   Miles journeyed: _____

Exercise chosen: _____

Spiritual thoughts: _____

_____

_____

_____

Feelings: _____

_____

_____

_____

16 The Difference between Heart Health and Weight Loss

BIBLICAL BIG IDEA #16

Your eye is the lamp of your body. If your eye is healthy, your whole body is full of light; but if it is not healthy, your body is full of darkness. —Luke 11:34

Several years ago, I had a huge "a-ha" moment regarding the difference between heart health and weight loss. For example, 10,000 steps per day is a great goal for heart health. This sort of activity level is ensuring that you are moving enough in the day to remain active and provide good perfusion (i.e., your heart is pumping blood to all parts of your body) to your cardio-respiratory system so that the heart continues to beat effectively. A strong and healthy heart is central to good health and longevity. A heart that beats strongly and sends oxygen-rich blood to all parts of the body helps to remove toxins, deliver healing properties to the body, boost the immune system, and build a body that is full of good health.

If you have never been active, a 10,000-step program may help you with weight loss. Depending on your current lifestyle and nutritional choices, a change towards 10,000 steps in a day could definitely be a good first step in a weight-loss plan. However, most people do not obtain the weight loss they seek with only a 10,000 step plan. Most individuals will need to boost their 10,000 steps to a 12,000- to 15,000-step plan to see weight-loss results. Ten thousand steps a day is really good for heart health. However, when trying to lose weight, we will often need to take physical activity to an even higher level to get the results we want. You will also need to look at your diet and begin removing all the processed junk from your pantry. Weight loss is a result of increased exercise and proper nutritional choices.

Remember, Christ Walk is not a diet; it is a way of living. However, I would be negligent in not addressing the weight-loss aspect of Christ

Walk as I realize that many people choose to start any exercise program in the hopes of losing weight. I am also very aware from my own experiences and the experience of others that it can be very frustrating to think that all you need to do to lose weight is move more, and then not see the results you were hoping for.

Weight loss occurs when you burn more calories than you put in your mouth. It takes a deficit of 3,500 calories in order to burn one pound of body weight. If the average individual requires 2,000 calories a day to maintain his or her weight, then that individual would have to cut 500 calories a day from his or her diet in order to lose one pound per week. Then, they would have to burn 500 calories additionally in a day to burn a total of two pounds a week. It takes a LOT of work, and a LOT of diligence, to lose weight. It means being vigilant and HONEST about every little thing you put in your mouth and everything you ask your body to do. The body is a complex machine. It needs the right kind of food and nutrients to burn fat in the most efficient way possible. This is why I recommend a diet of real food. In theory you could eat a low-caloric diet of junk food, but you probably wouldn't see the results you desired because it is not real food. Real food comes from God's earth. It is important to ensure that your food choices come from a wide variety of healthy sources. Your body needs to get a variety of nutrients from a variety of different sources in order to perform at an optimum level. Even if all we ate were bag after bag of carrots, the body would start to have problems, because that much vitamin A would be toxic. The body would also not be getting the variety of carbohydrates, protein, and fats that it needs to function well. Not only do you need to consider intake versus output (how many calories you put in versus how many calories you burn), you also need to make sure that the calories are quality calories that the body needs.

With our modernized food sources, processed carbohydrates and sugars are inserted into everything. High fructose corn syrup (HFCS) is an unnecessary additive to food that may not change the caloric intake of a processed food, but will add a completely unnecessary component to your diet. Other sugars are also added to many foods that can cause weight gain or can make losing weight extremely difficult. If you are finding it difficult to lose weight, make sure you are tracking the amount of sugar you may knowingly or unknowingly be adding to your diet. Drinks and packaged foods are the number-one culprits of adding unnecessary fillers to our diet. If you eat a real diet of real food from God's earth, you will be cutting many unnecessary additives from your life and you may see the results you seek in your weight loss.

A 10,000-step program might help you burn an extra 300 calories in a day, but if you are eating those extra calories, then it will not do your weight loss any good. It will be GREAT for your heart that you continue to move, but if your additional goal is to lose weight and change your body, you will have to make additional changes and sacrifices.

These guidelines can be overwhelming at first. It may be daunting to track calories and expenditure. However, if you are not writing down everything you put in your mouth, you are not aware of it. You may choose to use a pen and paper tracker to record your intake. Or, there are a number of smart phone apps available today that will help you track this for free. "My Fitness Pal" and "Lose It" are two examples of apps to track your intake. Not only do they calculate your required calories, but they also will help you identify where the high caloric foods are in your diet and steer you towards healthier choices. Research has shown that online communities help us to meet our goals. We can join groups that send us cheers on our exercise, or other groups in which people can compete for the number of steps in a day.

There are different apps, social media groups, and other computer communities that can help you reach your goal and keep you motivated. Sometimes we have an easier job being accountable to online groups. Some people will do better if they meet face to face. Either way, there are many options available to you to build that community of health and fitness. Hopefully, your church will be one of those communities of health as well!

Another reason that a 10,000-step program is often not sufficient to lose weight is that we hit plateaus when taking on exercise and nutritional changes. A plateau is when we hit a point where we cannot see change, either in the scale, measurement tape, speed, capability, or fit of clothes. The human body gets too comfortable with established routines when it comes to exercise. This means we need to make it sit up and listen by changing up our routine. This can include adding different exercises, increasing intensity/resistance to the workout we are doing, making additional healthy changes to our diet, or adding another 2,000 steps to our goal. Variety is the spice of life. Variety is the spice of exercise!

We also get complacent spiritually if we get too comfortable with established routines. As an Episcopalian, liturgical routines are a part of the norm for me. I must stay vigilant in my prayer and worship so that I am spiritually present in the moment and not just saying the words and motions from memory. I also enjoy trying new prayers and styles of church services so that my mind is always engaged. These are examples of switching it up.

With physical exercise, if you are not seeing changes with increased activity and decreased intake, it may be that your metabolism runs slower than the average, and you may need fewer calories than average. If your caloric needs are only 1,500 calories a day and you have based your caloric reduction on a 2,000 calorie diet, then you are not going to see the results you want; you will actually only be maintaining your calorie needs. A slow metabolism may be a sign of some other underlying metabolic problem that you should have checked. If you have the option available to you, I highly recommend that you seek out a wellness center or nutrition counselling center (or even your healthcare provider) to see if they can complete any testing to tell you your actual caloric needs. This will be much more useful to you in determining what you need for your body than guessing. Not only is it important to ensure you are reducing your calories sufficiently, you also need to ensure you are eating enough. Not eating enough can slow your metabolism and set you back in your goals. Finding your metabolic rate will help you discover this.

The pursuit of a healthy body is like being a Christian. Health and a healthy body are the pursuits of a lifetime. We need to constantly move and stay active to keep our bodies healthy. Likewise, as Christians we are called to constantly evolve ourselves in what we can do and give back to the world. I have never been comfortable that my life as a Christian was only about grace. My salvation, grace, and the forgiveness of my sins are from God alone. I cannot be made whole through my works alone. I cannot find forgiveness on my works alone; it is only through God's grace that I have the hope of salvation. However, once I accepted God's grace in my life, I do not believe that gives me the right to sit back and let things happen. My dad brought me up with the saying that "A faith without works is no faith." I have faith in God's forgiveness, grace, and healing in my life, but I will not be able to be the change in the world that God plans for me if I do nothing. Likewise, while I know that through his grace he gives me the strength to transform my body and my thoughts and my spirit, if I am not actively participating in the journey, I am not sure that it would bear the fruit I seek.

When you hit that plateau and are extremely frustrated that nothing is happening on the scale, or in your health, or on the trail—say a little prayer, love yourself as a gift from God, and think about what you might have to do next to build the temple as strong as you see it. Make sure that your vision of the temple is also God's vision. We are not all called to be models or actors and society's visions of a healthy temple. If you are active, healthy, and maintaining your temple, it may just be time to love the temple God gave you and do the work that he's called you to do with what you have. Sometimes our temple is healthy and working well, but it is our own discontent with ourselves that calls us to pursue a different body than the one God gave us. God will love you any way you look. And I can guarantee that as long as you are taking care of your body, nurturing it and loving it, your spirit will bloom no matter how you look. People around you will be drawn to your spirit first, not your outside shell. People will think you are amazing just as you are.

THOUGHTS TO PONDER

1. Do I need to lose weight, or do I need to focus on heart health?

2. What is my calorie intake (write it ALL down!)?

3. What is my calorie output? Am I burning 3,500 extra calories in a week to lose weight if that is my goal?

4. Am I eating the RIGHT kind of foods? Or is my calorie intake all junk food or fake diet food?

5. Does losing weight really need to be my goal?

6. What can I do this week to take my Christ Walk to the next level?

7. How do I see my current body? Is it strong enough to do God's work in the world?

O Lord, by these things people live, and in all these is the life of my spirit. Oh, restore me to health and make me live! —Isaiah 38:16

DAY 16 Steps taken: _____ Miles journeyed: _____

Exercise chosen: _____

Spiritual thoughts: _____

_____

_____

_____

Feelings: _____

_____

_____

_____

What Does the Bible Say about Food?

BIBLICAL BIG IDEA #17

On the banks, on both sides of the river, there will grow all kinds of trees for food. Their leaves will not wither nor their fruit fail, but they will bear fresh fruit every month, because the water for them flows from the sanctuary. Their fruit will be for food, and their leaves for healing. —Ezekiel 47:12

Ah, food, one of my favorite topics. I love food. I often joke that I will always exercise so that I can enjoy food. This is true. Exercise is good for my body, but it also gives me a little more leeway to enjoy some of my favorite foods with less guilt. Genesis is very clear that the fruit of the earth was given to us for food:

God said, "See, I have given you every plant yielding seed that is upon the face of all the earth, and every tree with seed in its fruit; you shall have them for food. And to every beast of the earth, and to every bird of the air, and to everything that creeps on the earth, everything that has the breath of life, I have given every green plant for food." And it was so. —Genesis 1:29–30

Oh, boy. This excites me! I love food from the earth. This is real food. I love REAL food. I have yet to find the biblical quote that teaches to "eat from the tree of meal replacement bars!" God did not say, "I give you low-fat, light, high fructose corn syrup, artificially colored, with a flavored nutritional substitute!" God gave us real food to eat. I am perplexed that we would choose anything else.

We have a bountiful selection of grains, fruits, vegetables, and meat to choose from. Over the years food has become even more plentiful and easier to access. For the first time in history, we really do not have to work for our food. It can be found wherever we turn. Where we have poverty of food in America, we have poverty of quality food. There is good food that is not fast food, processed, or from a box that we need to share with each other and with those that are without. Food is good for you. Food can heal. Food from the earth is healthy. Real food is a good thing and we should not be ashamed to eat real food and enjoy it.

Unfortunately, being humans, we have managed to mess that up as well. We have love/hate relationships with food. We turn to food for comfort rather than fuel; we use food to fill voids in our souls that food cannot fix. We use food as a reward, and we have forgotten what real hunger feels like because of the glut of food around us. We eat because we *think* we need to eat, not necessarily because we actually *need* to eat. Breakfast comes at 8:00 a.m., lunch at noon, and dinner at 6:00 p.m. without us actually listening to our bodies to tell us, "I am hungry now!"

On top of this, we move food great distances to get to our table. When food moves great distances, it means that it has been picked before it is ripe and left to ripen in a crate. Food that does not ripen on its plant is less nutritious and healthy for the body. This process reduces the nutrients (vitamins and minerals) in foods, and while we have more food than ever, the food is not as healthy for us as it has been in times past.

Added to the transportation and globalization of food, the industrialization of food products has added unnecessary additives and preservatives in the name of comfort and safety. We really do not know the implications of all this extra stuff in our food, but with the growing rates of obesity, diabetes, cancer, food allergies, and high blood pressure, it is easy to assume that there is a connection in what we eat, how we eat, and what it is doing to our bodies.

Industrialization of food began in order to ensure that a cheap and robust food supply was available for a growing population. This movement also spawned convenience foods, as fewer and fewer individuals were growing their own food supply as they moved closer to the city. Convenience foods were marketed as either fast foods to eat on the go, or as boxed products to make the "mom job" of cooking easier. These foods were also a huge part of marketing to the population as more women went back to work. When we are unable to till the earth ourselves, convenience and access to foods is important. However, we sacrificed healthy foods along the way to convenience. The truth about many convenience foods and "quick cooking" products is that it is not that much more difficult to make a recipe with real food than it is to rip open a box and mix in extra items. Advertising agencies don't want you to know this. The difference is you are able to control the additives and preservatives that you are introducing into your body when you make the choice for cooking real food for you and your family. In addition, genetically modified organism (GMOs) seeds are now used in the growing of many of the foods we eat.

The jury is out on the impact of GMOs on the body. Whenever we try to play God with life (including human, animal, or plant life) it is never good for us. Personally and theologically, I am not a fan of GMOs.

As you begin reducing the number of convenience foods in your pantry, grocery shopping can become stressful and overwhelming. I have often walked into a grocery store and felt the need to turn around and leave from the overwhelming nature of trying to make the right healthy choices. It is difficult to know what a good product is off the shelf unless you take the time to read labels. When you make a habit of knowing the products you are willing to put into your body, however, it does become easier. I was originally dismayed by the cost of choosing organic products. However, I have found that the less I purchase packaged foods, the more money I have to devote to wholesome *real* food. Convenience foods and packaged products are really not as inexpensive as the marketing leads you to believe. However, as you make the change in your pantry, the initial cost difference can cause sticker shock. If cost is an issue, it is far better that you choose whatever fresh fruits and grains and vegetables that you can, rather than purchasing organic—but organic is going to be the better health choice. It is going to be a battle to weigh need versus cost to do the right thing. Whatever choice you make, at least make the choice to reduce the amount of packaged, processed food you eat. It's just not real food.

Farmers' markets are making a resurgence; getting access to fresh produce that is locally grown is getting easier every year. I love to shop at farmers' markets. I am not overwhelmed. The cost is either comparable or less than at the store; I love being outdoors to shop and visit and talk with the farmers; and I always know I am getting the best food for my table. Making these changes and choices is a process. As you make small choices and changes, each change towards healthier choices becomes easier. I started small and each year I get healthier and healthier with the choices I make. As a result, my family also gets healthier and healthier.

As I replaced my pantry items with real food, rather than food from a box, I was able to make more and more food in my kitchen. I like to know that bread has just flour, yeast, water, salt, and oil in it, so I am more willing to make it myself. If I am going to eat chocolate cake, I want to know it has real butter, real sugar, real flour, and real eggs in it. I will offset this splurge by a smaller piece, but I will enjoy the cake far more knowing it is a real cake. If you look on the side of a box of cake mix, you will see far more items in the ingredients list than flour, sugar, and leavening. I do not want these additives in my body. If I am not able to make it myself, I am now more willing to spend a little more money to ensure that the best food product will make it into my kitchen.

When I look at my table after preparing a meal for my family, I feel joyful that I am able to give them the bounty from God's earth. Saying grace over a meal has added meaning when I know that the food is from God. I can joyfully celebrate knowing the food that I have selected came from the earth, not a processing plant. I also know that the food is better for me and my family. We all feel healthier. Our bodies feel great when we are fed from the earth. We do not get sick as often and our energy levels are high.

I know that I am still eating foods that are more processed than I want or that are not directly from the farmer. That is life. Sometimes, I am unaware of how a food has been made so I begin to research it and make new food decisions. Industrialized food is sneaky. It is highly addictive and crafted to tantalize as many of the senses as it can, while sneaking ingredients into your body that are just as addictive as nicotine or other drugs. Do not be fooled that food cannot act as a drug in your body. The process of bringing healthier foods to the table is just that, a process. I did not clean out my pantry overnight. I am sure that there are things I can still work on cutting out. I have made gradual changes so that each day is a better choice and each selection at the store or at the farmer's market is more a celebration of real food.

Real food makes me happy. I love to cook, I love to eat, and I love to share food with people. I look at it as a celebration of the gifts God gives us. Consider cutting one processed item from your house a week or a month, and slowly over the course of time you will see a healthier you. Your body will not crave the excess sugar and additives, your gut will be healthier, and your body will feel wonderful. Aches and pains will begin to disappear and you will get sick less often. You won't *see* these changes until you *start* making these changes in your food choices.

Jesus is ALWAYS eating in the Bible. Mealtimes were sacred. There was wine and bread and cheese and olives and meat. The food was prepared and shared in communion with family and friends so that relationships bloomed over food. People did not sit around obsessing if the broken bread would add an inch to their thighs. Food was a sacred and *joyful* experience. People ate joyfully all the time and they ate what they needed. They fasted when they needed to cleanse and center themselves. They were at peace with food. They were far more concerned about their relationship with God than with their relationship with food, and this is something that I think we can all learn. I am saddened that so many people have an unhappy relationship with food. Some people look at food as evil and it fills them with dread. If I could accomplish the task of bringing joy back into our relationship with food, then I think I will have accomplished something important.

My take on food is simple: get the best foods that you can that are as close to the earth as you can get them; eat when you are hungry, fast when you are not; and joyfully accept the bounty we have and share with those that do not.

THOUGHTS TO PONDER

1. How do I feel about food? Do I joyfully give thanks for the bounty that I have, or does food make me feel ashamed and guilty?

2. What does my pantry look like? Does it look like it came from an industrial plant? Or does it look like it came from the earth? Is the food as close to its natural state as I can find it? Or do I fill it with empty diet foods that are non-nutritious and do not fill the needs of my body?

3. What can I remove from my pantry today to make it cleaner and never go back?

4. How can I make mealtimes a joyful experience?

He humbled you by letting you hunger, then by feeding you with manna, with which neither you nor your ancestors were acquainted, in order to make you understand that one does not live by bread alone, but by every word that comes from the mouth of the LORD. —Deuteronomy 8:3

DAY 17   Steps taken: _____   Miles journeyed: _____

Exercise chosen: _____

Spiritual thoughts: _____

_____

_____

_____

Feelings: _____

_____

_____

_____

DAY 18 Tricks for More Exercise

BIBLICAL BIG IDEA #18

I shall walk at liberty, for I have sought your precepts.
—Psalm 119:45

Getting more exercise can be difficult for a number of reasons: life happens, injury happens, it is overwhelming, it is difficult to start something new, and many others. I have a self-defeating personality when it comes to a new exercise. The first thing I think as I try something new is, "I cannot do this." I start to be more concerned about what others think I can or cannot do and how I must look to others than putting God first in what I am doing.

When we are able to discard social dictates and secular rules to follow a Godly life, we are able to walk about freely. I find myself less concerned about the way I look and what others may say about me if I am trying to live a kindly and loving life.

For the whole law is summed up in a single commandment, "You shall love your neighbor as yourself." —Galatians 5:14

When I know that I am walking for others first, my baggage falls off and my walk is freer. Through God's grace and forgiveness, I am able to let go of self recriminations of what I did not get done. I know that if I continue to get up and walk with Christ, I have a new day, each day, to try again.

Every day I will bless you, and praise your name forever and ever. —Psalm 145:2

Walking with Christ is a forever event.

Unfortunately, I am human. I fail to remember to walk with Christ daily. I find it easy to forget to talk to God about my fears. I start living on my own and having relationships more about me than us (Christ and myself). I begin to worry if I am thin enough, good-looking enough, fast enough, smart enough, or whatever it may be; I become paralyzed by self-centeredness. When my life is about me, me, me, I am miserable. We are called to be there for others first, and my Christ Walk needs to be about me being the best I can be for what God has called me to do.

I believe a healthy body is a part of what God has called me to do. I believe that taking care of this physical form for as long as we have it is a godly thing to do. We should love it and care for it and not abuse it and fill it with harmful things and harmful actions.

Glorify God in your body. —1 Corinthians 6:20b

When it comes to taking care of the body with physical exercise, things happen. Remember, it can be hard to start something new. It may be that life gets in the way of your goal; illness, a death in your family, disability, work, or social obligations may intrude on your well-developed plan. These "life events" over which you have no control can feel very defeating if you let them. Using a pedometer to monitor your physical exercise can be one method of ensuring you get exercise, even around these life events. I love wearing a pedometer because it gives me an idea of how much I am really moving my body on the days where I am running around like a chicken, but not getting any formal exercise. The pedometer can tell me if I need to move more or if all my running around was more exercise than I thought. I also use a pedometer to sneak in extra exercise as a part of a normal day. Every time we use the stairs, park farther away, go for a ten-minute power walk, or get up to move is an opportunity to sneak in exercise. These are ways to add movement into my day without necessarily carving out an hour of my day to do it.

My tricks for getting in those extra steps and extra miles vary. First, I always try to park as far away from my destination as I can to add those steps. I never have to fight for a parking space at the back of a parking lot. Instead of getting everything I need from upstairs, I do one thing at a time so that I have to make multiple trips up and down the stairs. I often take out one item out of the dishwasher at a time so that I have to walk that much farther to get the chore done. I include yard work and cleaning as a part of my exercise. Every hour I get up from my desk and walk around or do sit ups, jumping jacks, push-ups, squats, or lunges for five minutes. If I do this at least five to eight times in a work day, then I have squeezed in a top to bottom strength workout without having to go anywhere. I can always find five minutes to do this, but rarely can find an hour on crazy days.

I like to walk my kids to school (or bike them) and we have always tried to live close enough to town amenities that they are in walking or biking distance. I dislike driving, so I enjoy being able to bike or walk on my errands whenever possible. We also tend to build our family outings around a physical activity such as hiking, sailing, putt-putt, skating, bowling, and other physical adventures so that we are moving and having fun at the same time. Finally, when I cannot get in my normal workout, I often try to take short walks at multiple times during the day so that I am at least doing something. It is better to do fifteen minutes of something than a whole day of nothing. Then the next day you can try for something longer or harder. Always try to move daily.

The whole point of a healthy lifestyle is to build it into your own daily routine. We do not pick and choose the times to be Christian, we do not (or should not) limit our Christian duties and actions to Sunday morning. Rather, the actions and choices we make should be a part of how we live our life daily. Sneaking in exercise should not sound sneaky; it should be a way of thinking. How can I move more today when life is happening and I am not sure that my normal routine will happen? We should live our lives thinking, "How can I pray more and talk more to God? How can I make God a little more of my life and how I live today?" Exercise, eating right, praying, loving, joyous actions, study, and kindness are about a lifestyle, not a schedule. How will you choose to live your life healthier today?

THOUGHTS TO PONDER

1. How can I change my life today to live healthier?

2. What can I do daily to add more physical activity to my life?

3. Do I look at my healthy actions as something to be scheduled? Or am I living a LIFESTYLE of Christian behavior? How can I do it better?

His divine power has given us everything needed for life and godliness, through the knowledge of him who called us by his own glory and goodness.
—2 Peter 1:3

DAY 18   Steps taken: _____   Miles journeyed: _____

Exercise chosen: _____

Spiritual thoughts: _____

_____

_____

_____

_____

Feelings: _____

_____

_____

_____

_____

Living in Reality:
"Christ Walk" for Where
You Are Now

BIBLICAL BIG IDEA #19
When you walk, your step will not be hampered; and if you run,
you will not stumble. —Proverbs 4:12

Just as there are days where we need to exercise more and overcome our
innate laziness, there are also days when we need to listen to our bodies
and do what we can do. Some days may not be exercise of the body days,
but may be exercise of the spirit and soul days through prayer, meditation, and fasting. There is a time and a place for everything. What we
need to do is listen to our bodies and become attuned to their needs so
we are treating our bodies well.

I had a very difficult time the last several years coming to terms with
my running. If I am honest about it, I do like running, although it is a
bit of a love/hate relationship. I do not feel that I am very good at running and it is extremely hard on my body to run long distances. Despite
many visits to physicians and experts, no one can quite figure out why
I have so many problems when I run a long distance. I struggle with
gastrointestinal and urinary problems when I run long distance and no
test can find anything wrong. I began to feel that the longer I was running (even following training regimens safely with expert guidance), the
more I was hurting my body. I had to come to a decision that perhaps
right now was not the time for me to run distance. Rather, I needed to
heal my body first.

I do not think my race days are over, but again, I came to a realization
that in the balance of my life, I needed to put distance running aside and
heal my body, take care of my family, and focus on what I can do that will
also keep me healthy. I often get frustrated because I feel that unless I am
doing extreme exercise, then I won't be able to maintain my weight or

stay at my ideal level of fitness. This has led me to realize I need to love myself wherever I am in this moment in life because it is only a moment. Even though I may not be looking like a scion of health, it does not mean that I cannot still share my gifts that God has given to me at this moment in time. Where we are in time is not stagnant and will always change.

When I could love myself at this moment, the burden of how I exercised and why I exercised began to change. It stressed me out less not to be exercising at my maximum capacity, but rather to enjoy the walk that I was on at that point in my life. As my body begins to heal and I feel rejuvenated and more wholesome, I do realize that one day, when it is the right time and place, I can take up distance running again. I am okay with this. There is a time and a place for everything.

During my mother's bone marrow transplant treatment, she was in the hospital for about three or four weeks undergoing the main part of her treatment. Obviously, she was not running any marathons (nor will she ever) at that point in her life. Mom's Christ Walk during her treatment was to put five pennies in the window outside her hospital room and pick one up each time she walked a lap around the wing of the hospital. Her goal was to do five laps each day; each penny reminded her how many she needed to go per day. My mom walked to stave off boredom, keep moving, push herself past depression and self pity, stay stronger, help with the pain and nausea, and remind herself that she was not defined by her cancer. When my mom walked through her treatment, her walk reminded my mom that her life was not the four corners of her hospital room. Getting out of her hospital room allowed her to see that there were other lives on the floor that were happening at the same time and not just her own story. By looking outside of her own grief and seeing others, my mom was better able to handle the stress of her own illness.

When we are able to see outside of ourselves, we move past the sin of self-centeredness. Then our story on earth is not about the self, but about us: our relationships with each other.

Do nothing from selfish ambition or conceit, but in humility regard others as better than yourselves. Let each of you look not to your own interests, but to the interests of the others. —Philippians 2:3–4

By making her walk about more than herself, my mom lifted Christ into her illness and was able to Christ Walk through the dark moments of her life. This was my mom's Christ Walk at that time and place in her life. Your Christ Walk will change at different points in your life and it is all okay. There is a time and a place for everything.

There is a time and a place for all kinds of Christ Walks in life, and your Christ Walk changes every day, every year, every month, and every moment. The purpose of your Christ Walk is to never stop walking with Christ. If today is not the day that you will walk your journey, then give yourself and your heart over to God so that the relationship continues. There are many illnesses, diseases, infirmities, social strictures, and societal norms that say, "You can't." I believe in saying, "Yes you can," no matter what. You can always do something. It may be small. It may not be the distance, the race, or the effort that you imagined. But as long as you are doing something and God is there with you while you are doing it, you are making your temple stronger. It is all a matter of what you believe and how much you are willing to let your imagination flourish.

Christ Walk for today, not tomorrow or yesterday. Learn to do what you can and not burden yourself with the negative thinking patterns of what you cannot.

There are hundreds of races, walks, and bike rides now for people who have been told, "You can't" because of something that might have happened to them. They have chosen to say, "Yes, I CAN." This is an attitude that resonates with me. Life happens, but the journey does not stop. Crossroads in life rarely have stop signs that say, "No more." You have to figure out how you will go on in your journey when life happens. You will need to accept what your Christ Walk will be for today—and then do that.

I am the queen of self-recriminating comments about how slow I run, how I could do better, how I should be faster, fitter, thinner, prettier, holier, you name it. I can beat myself up and down the road over "Shoulda, woulda, coulda." This does not do anyone good: not me, not my family, not my friends, and not the things I need to do for others. These thoughts make it all about me and less about doing what I need to do to stay strong enough for the call I have in this world. When I am occupied about thoughts of the self, I am not living in the moment. No matter how poorly I have run the race, I can still proclaim joyfully that God was there with me through it all. In every moment, God is with me in that Christ Walk, and if I am not joyfully sharing that moment, then it has turned back to being about me and not about this relationship with God that I am trying to nurture. I do not believe that there is ever a day that we cannot do something. It may not be what we thought we could do that day, or be called to do, but it will be something. Even on the day we die, we have that choice to live with the angels, the archangels, and all the company of heaven, gloriously singing the praises of God.

The question is: Will you choose to proclaim God no matter where you are on your Christ Walk?

THOUGHTS TO PONDER

1. Am I Christ Walking today, at my ability level, and sharing the journey with God?

2. Do I need to rethink my Christ Walk for this day and moment in my life?

3. What do I need to let go of on my journey so that I am not being self-defeating?

Then Esau said, "Let us journey on our way, and I will go alongside you."
—Genesis 33:12

DAY 19   Steps taken: _____   Miles journeyed: _____

Exercise chosen: _____

Spiritual thoughts: _____

_____

_____

_____

Feelings: _____

_____

_____

_____

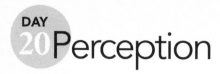

DAY 20 Perception

BIBLICAL BIG IDEA 20

*One dies in full prosperity, being wholly at ease and secure,
his loins full of milk, and the marrow of his bones moist.
Another dies in bitterness of soul, never having tasted
of good.* —Job 21:23–25

About one-third of all Americans are considered obese according to national health standards. Your favorite football or basketball player may be obese by these measures, as obesity is calculated on the body mass index (BMI), which is a ratio between your weight in kilograms and your height in meters (squared). The formula is used because most people who are heavy have a corresponding high ratio of body fat on their frames. This formula actually does not take into consideration one's muscular makeup when defining obesity versus normal weight. Muscle weighs more than fat. Therefore heavily muscled individuals can actually be considered obese on the BMI scale.

This does not mean we throw away years of obesity research on questionable math. My belief is that it is not all about the numbers. You can have a skinny person who does not take care of him- or herself, has no cardio-respiratory endurance, and may be just as unhealthy as someone who is heavier and denser but takes care of his or her body. I have a friend who used to jokingly say, "Have you ever seen a fat alcoholic?" And if you think about it, there are few overweight alcoholics, but that does not mean they are healthy. On the contrary, the excessive drinking is just as damaging to the body as excessive eating.

Unfortunately, Americans on a whole are becoming victims to the rich and bounteous lifestyle that has grown from our economic success. We have discussed the abundance and accessibility of food, the wonders of transportation and modern gadgets that make life easier, and how the nature of life has become more and more sedentary, lending ourselves to a portlier lifestyle. The fact of the matter is, no matter how BMI/obesity is calculated, we all have some work to do in maintaining the health God gave us. Every day, we *all* have the opportunity to make better choices towards better health.

Most individuals grossly underestimate the amount of calories they eat and grossly overestimate the amount of physical activity that they do. Men are more likely to see themselves in a mirror and think they look pretty good while women are more likely to see themselves as a lot worse than they are. It seems to me that none of us are very good at judging ourselves with our own eyes. My mother used to tell me that my eyes were always bigger than my stomach, and it is true. And when my eyes are bigger than my stomach, my backside gets bigger than my britches. Unless you are measuring and weighing and mindful of what you are doing, you probably are way off the mark in how much you are taking in compared to burning off. Our perception rarely reflects reality.

We also do not have a good sense of what we look like. Our self-critical perceptions mislead us in how the world perceives us. I know that I perceive myself differently based on mood alone. One day I can look in the mirror and be satisfied by what I see and on other days my perception reflects an individual with different shapes and different capabilities. If I let my self-centeredness dwell on the image in the mirror, I am not focusing on what this temple can do with the tools God gave it.

Our perceptions can be faulty. It can be discouraging to be told you are overweight when you may have very strong cardio-respiratory fitness. It can be very discouraging each day to look in the mirror and let self-defeating words beat down the image you see. It can be discouraging to take on a new practice towards a healthy lifestyle not knowing where you really are and where you really need to go. However, you can take care of the temple God gave you. Move away from the perception of what size and shape you should be and focus on accomplishing the things you can do to make your body stronger to accomplish your goals.

This is when it is really good to talk to some experts in the field. Invest in a fitness test that will not only tell you what your weight is, but also your body fat, BMI, strength, cardiovascular fitness level, flexibility, blood pressure, and resting heart rate. These are all components of a healthy temple. By assessing these components of fitness, you can receive an objective measurement of what your body is capable of doing. As you walk more frequently and become more active, these measurements of cardiovascular fitness will improve. Hopefully, these numbers will help you to see yourself as a healthy temple, even if it is not some image you have set for yourself. I have a doctor friend who likes to say that if your pants still fit the same over the last ten years, you can still walk a couple of miles without getting winded, and are able to do your activities of daily living with vigor, then you are probably doing pretty well. Not all of us are created to be athletes, and not all of us are created to be models. We all, however, have been given bodies that will do the work of God in the world if we take care of them and keep them fit. Our energy should be directed to taking care of our bodies and using these bodies towards God's will.

Chapter 21 in the book of Job speaks so strongly to this. If you do not experience the good and joyful in what can be done with yourself as you are, you will die bitter, probably unable to reconcile yourself and your relationship with Christ. This is a great sin. Rather, we should live vigorously and joyfully with our relationship with God and what we are called to do. Do not let your perceptions get in the way of what is real and right.

One of my favorite prayers that helps me center myself for a balanced way of living is "A Morning Resolve" from Forward Movement Publications. This prayer is so incredibly powerful to me as it helps me to organize my life around mind, body, and spiritual health and it is about living in today:

> I will try this day to live a simple, sincere and serene life, repelling promptly every thought of discontent, anxiety, discouragement, impurity, and self-seeking; cultivating cheerfulness, magnanimity, charity, and the habit of holy silence; exercising economy in expenditure, generosity in giving, carefulness in conversation, diligence in appointed service, fidelity to every trust, and a childlike faith in God.
>
> In particular I will try to be faithful in those habits of prayer, work, study, physical exercise, eating, and sleep, which I believe the Holy Spirit has shown me to be right. And as I cannot in my own strength do this, nor even with a hope of success attempt it, I look to thee, O Lord God my Father, in Jesus my Savior, and ask for the gift of the Holy Spirit.*

If there was ever one prayer that conveys my thoughts, feelings, and beliefs about living a Christ Walk–centered life, this is that prayer. When I pray this prayer, it reminds me—live in peace. I pray that I live my life the best way I can, in the way the Holy Spirit has shown me to be right. When I have balanced my mind, body, and spiritual health in the Holy Spirit, all is right with my world. When I am balanced in my mind, body and spiritual health, my worries do not plague me. Then I am stepping my Christ Walk in tune with the Lord, and those are really good days.

---

*Used with permission by Forward Movement. This prayer is offered in each issue of the daily devotional, "Forward Day by Day."

THOUGHTS TO PONDER

1. What are my perceptions about myself?

2. Are these the same as how others see me?

3. Do I need to get some objective measures of my health and fitness? Who can I talk to? Will this help me to move towards a healthier life?

For from the greatness and beauty of created things comes a corresponding perception of their Creator. —Wisdom of Solomon 13:5

DAY 20   Steps taken: _____   Miles journeyed: _____

Exercise chosen: _____

Spiritual thoughts: _____

_____

_____

_____

Feelings: _____

_____

_____

_____

Christ Walk Moms

BIBLICAL BIG IDEA #21
Blessed is the womb that bore you and the breasts that nursed you! —Luke 11:27

Rather than talk about myself as a mom, I would like to tell you about my own mother and the other mothers in my life who have taught me a little something about being a mom. These moms have shown me through their actions how to Christ Walk as a mom.

First, there was my grandmother Neenie. She died about six weeks after I married my husband. She was not your traditional grandmother who baked cookies and sent lavish presents. Rather, my grandmother taught me how to plant a garden (although I have a brown thumb). She taught me how to cook the most amazing roast you will ever eat and make the best squash pie (even my own mother cannot make Neenie's squash pie—sorry, Mom). Above all, Neenie taught me how important the gift of time is to my children. She taught me about the fruits of the earth and the comfort of food.

My other grandmother, Deeda, was very involved in politics in South Carolina. For a woman of the 1950's, she was very vocal and active in her community. Being a female active in politics at that time was not always the social norm. She was opinionated about her beliefs and was not afraid to share them. I come by being opinionated naturally. But whether you call it being overly opinionated or standing up for what you believe in, my grandmother Deeda taught me that it is important to have beliefs and share them. Passing on a set of beliefs helps to identify your values. One's beliefs set the stage for the development of lifelong passions and skills that go with you wherever you may be. Our beliefs and how we share them will shape the world for the future. The courage to "be the change you want to see in the world" is such a valuable lesson to share with generations to come. The world will not change if we sit back and do nothing.

Then there is my mother-in-law, Sandra. When I hear friends complain about their mothers-in-law, I count my blessings. My mother-in-law is a wonderful role model. Not only can she cook, but she can organize and plan and take care of any disaster. Sandra left little bitty Bowman, South Carolina, to go to big, bad Washington, DC, to be the personal secretary for Senator Strom Thurmond when she was in her twenties. She applied for the job at the urging of her own mother, who thought it would be cool to have a rejection letter from Senator Thurmond. This woman is fierce. She is a determined woman both personally and professionally. I cannot begin to tell you the strength of will and love for her family that this woman has. I am convinced that my mother-in-law has a pipeline to God. When she prays about something, God sits up and listens. She has shown me how important family is not only to her, but also to me. Wherever we go in the world, I know that we have a welcome in her home in South Carolina that will always be ours to share. This gift of family is something for me to pass on to my kids. Her amazing discipline for prayer is one I strive for each day.

My girlfriends—who else could I call when I was nursing my babies in the middle of the night and was sure they were going to die because I had no idea how much food they were getting? Who else was I to call in tears when my son and I fought for the first time? Who else do you call when you aren't sure that you are doing something right, but desperately need to hear that the best job you are doing is a great job? My girlfriends are the gift of friends that I want to pass on to my children.

And I would not be a mom without my husband. He makes me a better mom through his support and love and encouragement. I sometimes think he is the better parent! If only he could cook! He gives me the time to write Christ Walk and to run. Working together we make our house a Christ-centered home to raise our children. Without my husband, I would stumble in my call to be a parent.

Finally, there is my own mother. She is an amazing woman. While I have always grown up within a church and while my dad taught us about churches—it was my mom that taught me about faith. While I was losing my hearing and my father was ill, my mother was there. If there was a backbone that kept my family together in the midst of this turmoil, it was my mother. She had to juggle my health, my dad's health, my brother leaving for school, my father's discharge from the Navy, and our family's move from Rhode Island to South Carolina. This period of my life is one I will always remember as the most turbulent. It is a bond that I share with my mother like no other. She drove me through a snow storm—a blizzard that stretched from Rhode Island to Ohio (where we were headed) to try to get me to a specialist to stop my hearing loss. She prayed a lot. A LOT! And I remember years later talking about this time with my mom and asking her how she continued to go to church through all this, and she said it was her faith in God that would get her through this time. And it did. My mom's quiet, serene faith (she would laugh if she heard that), is something that I hold onto every day. This is the faith that I want to pass on to my children. The gift of faith is the most precious gift of them all.

If there was any gift I could give to moms, I would have to tell them it is important to take a little time for yourself. It is important to be healthy for you and your family—mind, body, and spirit. I used to agonize that I never seemed to have time for elaborate meditation or complex prayers of intercession, praise, and thanksgiving, but what I have learned is that in the busy times of your life, God loves the small prayers too. So I remind myself to say, "Praise God" and "Lord, I'm not sure what to pray for, but I know I need help" and "Thanks, God." Because I know that God knows the deepest petitions of my heart, the most heartfelt prayers can be simple and vague and but still understood. And that brings me peace.

Central to a life of Christ Walk is love. Central to any happy family is love. 1 John 4:7–21 teaches us to love one another. Christ Walking as a mom is teaching love.

Beloved, since God loved us so much, we also ought to love one another.
—1 John 4:11

This is the essential prerequisite in supporting Christian family well-being. Christ Walk moms build a house of faith for their families by being moms.

If a widow has children or grandchildren, they should first learn their religious duty to their own family and make some repayment to their parents; for this is pleasing in God's sight. —1 Timothy 5:4

So, today, I pray that all of us mothers will indeed have God's help and God's love in us, so that we are able to promote an environment of love in our families.

If you are not yet a mother, or will not be a mother, the beliefs you hold and how you present yourself can also be shared with younger generations. We all have children that look up to us, no matter our role in their lives. Share the values and beliefs you received from your mother, or your female role models, with the children around you. They will only be lifted up by your care.

For all the women in my life, I give thanks to God. For all the women who are taking the Christ Walk journey for health for them and their families, I pray for perseverance. And for all the mothers who are living the life of faith for their children, I give praise. Amen.

THOUGHTS TO PONDER

1. Do you see your role as parent as a calling from God?

2. How do you feel about balancing what you need to do for your health with the health of your family and their needs?

3. What helps you find this balance?

4. If you are not a parent, do you see a role for yourself in leading the little children?

Honor your father and your mother, so that your days may be long in the land that the LORD your God is giving you. —Exodus 20:12

DAY 21 Steps taken: _____   Miles journeyed: _____

Exercise chosen: _____

Spiritual thoughts: _____

_____

_____

_____

Feelings: _____

_____

_____

_____

The Grocery Store

BIBLICAL BIG IDEA #22

*And also take with you every kind of food that is eaten, and
store it up; and it shall serve as food for you and for them.*
—Genesis 6:21

The grocery store: a house of plenty or a place of temptation? I hate going
to the grocery store, which is pretty amazing considering how much I
love food. I love to explore food, create food, cook food, and experiment
with food. I love to go to farmers' markets, outdoor markets, berry farms,
and gourmet food stores. If I had money to burn, I would not think twice
about where I shopped for food. However, my pocketbook constrains me
on where I can shop for food. My work and life schedules influence where
I spend my time looking for food. If we lived thirty years ago, we would
spend more time and money investing in food. Unfortunately, I have to
live in the world that I have created for myself, and so I do not have the
time to shop around at a million places, or spend a lot of money on gourmet food. I have to work within the limits of my life, and that means the
grocery store.

(Groan.)

The best advice I was given about the grocery store is to stay on the
outside aisles. This is great advice. If you hit the outside and load up
on the fruits, vegetables, dairy, and meats/fish and avoid the processed
mess in the middle aisles, you are doing pretty well. The middle aisles
are temptation—the yummy, addictive, processed goodness (but bad for
you) creations that were created for the very means of making your body
think you cannot live without it. Grocery stores place these foods stra-
tegically to force you to go through these aisles in order to make it from
the fresh produce down to the milk/butter/cheese/eggs area that we rely
on to make our own food. Grocery store creators know that if you have
to pass through these areas then you are more likely to stop and get the
salty/sweet/sour sensation that will be triggered by looking at the addictive packaging. Just writing and thinking about what the package of cook-

ies or chips looks like has my mouth salivating and sending signals to my brain that, "Ooooh, that sounds good," even when I am not hungry. These foods are designed to be as addictive as a drug and if you do not have the willpower to resist, I advise you to move away from these areas and avoid them at all costs.

Remember, it takes six months or longer to make a lifestyle change a habit. If you have not resisted your temptation for six months or longer, it is going to be really difficult to walk down the addicts' aisle and bypass your favorite junk food. And it is junk food. If you purge the junk and process out of your pantry and really detox your body from it, after time, you will not even crave it anymore. Over time, when you are not exposing yourself to a drug over and over again, you need it less. Over time, your body will no longer desire or crave these chemical substances. However, all of this takes time and persistence. Does this mean that the occasional junk food will harm you? I think the jury is out between various experts, but my take on things is that anything in moderation is probably okay. However, you have to know your addictions and weaknesses and ask yourself, "Will I really stop at one cookie (or whatever the serving size)?" Very few alcoholics or drug addicts can take just one drink or smoke and then walk away. Once they have given up their addiction, it's all or nothing. This is because drugs, tobacco, alcohol, and food for certain individuals *is* an addiction and the only way to overcome it is an all-or-nothing approach. Not all people have the same addictions. You will need to identify yours and decide where you will draw the line with it and then do not cross it.

Other things I hate about the grocery store—there is way too much stuff. There is way too much marketing of healthy items that probably are not healthy. There are so many misleading labels that you must read the fine print on the ingredient list. You will not know what you are putting into your body unless you read the list of components that make up the product. I also dislike the degree of variety in processed foods. Variety in plant and animal products is fantastic. Variety in manufactured food is a dangerous path. There are so many choices. This scares me because I go into information overload whenever I go to a grocery store. It becomes difficult to discern the healthy choice.

What I have learned to do is try to stick to the outside of the grocery store and run like a mad woman through what I *have* to get in the center aisles. I read the aisle headings before I head down any of them to ensure I do not track down the cookie aisle. If I am going to buy processed/prepared food, I will fork out the extra money to try to get the healthiest/least processed version available. I have learned to read labels and ask myself if I can make a better/healthier product on my own rather than buy it from the package. I avoid diet foods like the plague. I need to be satisfied by food, not filled by empty ingredients that leave me starving a couple of hours later because the diet food simply does not fill me with the nutrients my body needs. I like REAL food and I am far more willing to watch my portion sizes than I am to give up real cheese, real butter, or real sour cream just because it has fat in it.

These are the choices I chose to make. In order for me to enjoy the real food, I have to measure and check portion sizes. I use cups and measures to ensure that I am not putting a ¼ cup of dressing on my salad instead of the two teaspoons that is the actual portion size. I watch my calories. I sit at a computer most days writing, which is a sedentary, not active life. I must balance my intake (through calorie counting) with my sedentary lifestyle and look for ways to increase my activity. These are the things I have to do to keep my body healthy and working around the reality of my life.

You will have to figure out what you will need to do that works for you. You will need to start reading labels, measuring, deciding how to prepare food, and exploring the healthier options in produce and meat. In the summer, I hit the farmers' market because the selections are even better than the store (and keeps me away from that crazy building a little more). In the winter, I have fewer choices, but again, I do have choices. It just depends how I make them. The grocery store has many choices for you. You need to establish a plan before you enter it so that you are making the healthiest choice for you and your temple.

THOUGHTS TO PONDER

1. What are my frustrations with the grocery store?

2. What is one change I can make today in my pantry? (Write it down! Post a note on your pantry so you can see it every day! "The cookies have been banished! Have a piece of fruit! Or nuts! Or veggies!")

3. What choices can I make for a healthier meal/pantry?

4. How can I tame the grocery store instead of the grocery store taming me?

For every species of beast and bird, of reptile and sea creature, can be tamed and has been tamed by the human species. —James 3:7

DAY 22   Steps taken: _____   Miles journeyed: _____

Exercise chosen: _____

Spiritual thoughts: _____

_____

_____

_____

_____

Feelings: _____

_____

_____

_____

_____

PULSE CHECK JUDGMENT

Judgment is difficult to discuss. Judgment can mean many different things to different people. It can be a frightening word, or it can be a word filled with justice and truth, depending on your perspective. Justice can convey righted wrongs or harsh punishment. Judgment can feel unfair and unjustified. It is difficult to consider that things that happen in our life are a type of judgment based on our action by others or us.

Our culture is very judging. People pass judgment on each other about the way they look, the way they dress, and the way they act. People are quick to judge the actions without taking into consideration the context of individuals and their life experiences. We often look first at the splinter in another's eye without thinking of the log in our own. How well God knows us!

Judgment is valued in our society. People value the ideal that those who have done wrong will get what is due them. Many people secretly look at those with hard times in their lives and assume that they must have done something wrong that got them to this point.

"But you are obsessed with the case of the wicked; judgment and justice seize you." —Job 36:17

We are much more likely to assume individual responsibility for the outcomes in individual lives. "It must be that person's fault that got them there in the first place." "That person must have cancer because they did something wrong." Because our lives are short, we fail to consider that our actions as a society may affect the health and wellbeing of others in the future. Did the inclusion of high fructose corn syrup and GMOs in our food source contribute to the rise of chronic illnesses? Are these political choices now playing out in our health? Were these right or wrong choices? Were the results of these technological advances judgments on a societal decision? Our lives are short and it is difficult to say what is right or wrong with certainty. We blithely move through the world thinking it is ours, without considering that we need to take care of it for generations to come. We make many decisions in the world without knowing or understanding the long-term consequences of those decisions.

Judgment can be interpreted as a conflicting message between the Old Testament and the New Testament. We are brought up with the tradition that the God of the Old Testament is a God who delivers judgment and retribution with both hands:

When I whet my flashing sword, and my hand takes hold on judgment;
I will take vengeance on my adversaries, and will repay those who hate me.
—Deuteronomy 32:41

Whereas the God of the New Testament is one of love, light, and forgiveness:

You judge by human standards; I judge no one. —John 8:15

However, if we look closely at the Old Testament, we gain a deeper understanding of God:

I am the Lord, and I will free you from the burdens of the Egyptians and deliver you from slavery to them. I will redeem you with an outstretched arm and with mighty acts of judgment. —Exodus 6:6

and

You must not be partial in judging: hear out the small and great alike; you shall not be intimidated by anyone, for judgment is God's. Any case that is too hard for you, bring to me, and I will hear it. —Deuteronomy 1:17

and

Remember the wonderful works he has done, his miracles, and the judgments he uttered. —Psalm 105:5

The God of the Old Testament is not one without heart. God has not changed from Old Testament to New Testament; rather our understanding of God has evolved. In the New Testament, judgment continues,

The Father judges no one but has given all judgment to the Son. —John 5:22

and

Jesus said, "I came into this world for judgment so that those who do not see may see, and those who do see may become blind." —John 9:39

Throughout both the Old Testament and the New Testament, God is calling us not to judge others—to leave that work for God alone, and to focus on what we can do: love one another. Judgments help us to determine what is wrong. Judgments are sometimes the consequences of the world in which we live, the only way we can reconcile ourselves to those various judgments is through a loving relationship with God that seeks repentance and is open to reconciliation. This is true for our health as well. If you choose to look at your health problems as judgments on your body for things known and unknown, no matter how your prognosis goes, you always have the opportunity for reconciliation with God and that is more healing than any medicine in the world.

PART FOUR

REPENTANCE

Prayer

BIBLICAL BIG IDEA #23

Regard your servant's prayer and his plea, O LORD my God, heeding the cry and the prayer that your servant prays to you today. —1 Kings 8:28

As I look back over the last twenty-two days, I have come to realize that while I have talked about a lot of subjects and touched on the topic here and there, I have failed to devote some specific time to prayer. It is not because I have not thought about prayer, but because I look at prayer as weaved in through the context of everything I am doing for my health. Without prayer, I would be a sick, sick, sick soul. I feel physically ill when I have not been talking to God. I am acutely aware that there is something missing in my life when I have allowed myself to let that relationship with God flounder. There are times in my life when I have stepped off the path of walking with God to walking on my own and I know that something is out of step, but I am not sure how I got there or how to get back. I am immensely grateful that God seems to wait patiently for me each time to renew our relationship. I have found God to be greatly loving and welcoming no matter how many times I have done this or will continue to do this in my life.

I believe I will continue to have those moments of divergent walking because I have a tendency to believe that I can walk and work my life and not bother God with the details. I make a lot of assumptions about God's capabilities in my life (and you know what they say about assuming). I often tend to push God to the back of my consciousness when I get embroiled in something, thinking, "God, you are too busy for this pettiness." Invariably, when I try to handle things on my own, I end up running back, crawling back, or slinking back, with the thoughts, "I should have known better." I am human. I seem to make a lot of the same mistakes with my relationship with God and again; I am awed by God's grace that the door is never shut. God continues to forgive me and welcome me back with open arms. Each year, I gain a little wisdom to first say, "I cannot do this without you by my side."

Prayer is essential to a healthy life. There is a great deal of evidence of the health benefits of prayer and meditation on the body (Check out www.takingcharge.csh.umn.edu/explore-healing-practices/prayer for more in-depth information on the benefits of prayer and meditation). The rewards of prayer and meditation are huge. People who have an active prayer and/or meditation life have been shown to respond better to medical therapy when they present with acute or chronic diseases. Prayer and meditation have been used to help control high blood pressure, rapid heart rates, pain, anxiety and other physical symptoms. You can control a wide array of emotions and mental responses through prayer and meditation. Prayer and meditation tap into the biofeedback process that brings mindfulness to the physical form (or awareness to your body's responses). Prayer and meditation release endorphins for that "feel good" feeling, and provides the opportunity for personal insights. We often need to clear our brains first of our troubles before insights will occur on addressing these problems.

My notions about intentional prayer are a bit preconceived. I become a little cross-eyed at meal times because my children think that the best prayer to God for their food is "Bless our friends, bless our family, bless our food. Amen." If you think about it, this grace covers all the bases. However, as I try to guide my children in their spiritual lives, I am reminded that the way they think of God is different from the way I do, and I have to let their prayers be lifted up to God as they are. There will be a time for more elaborate grace in their lives, but I have to say, for now, this grace comes from their heart and that is a good thing.

Any prayer that comes from the heart is a good prayer, even if it is not memorized from a prayer book. I believe that any conversation with God is a prayer; even if it is not in a structured environment with standard words. I have the hardest time with a disciplined, structured prayer life. Making *time* that is dedicated to prayer is something I work on. I have to clear my mind of all the busyness of my life in order to focus on the words that I am saying. I have to work on bringing the *now* to my daily prayers. When I say the words of the Lord's Prayer, I have to call myself to focus and ask myself, "What am I saying?" Otherwise, coming from a liturgical background (which I love), I have a tendency for the prayers and actions of worship to become rote and business as usual. I am not fully present if I am not bringing my whole self to the table when working on my intentional prayers, and this for me is another aspect of my body and soul development. This form of prayer I must repeat and practice in order for it to become a part of my daily discipline. For some, intentional prayer comes easily; for others, they struggle as I do. But any prayer is good as long as you are working on your relationship with God as a part of it.

I practice intentional prayer just as any discipline, but I am far more inclined to have a continuous conversation with God. On my walks, in my work, and while driving my car I can take moments to talk with God. I want my heart open to share every aspect of my life with God, and I try to have a continuous conversation with God. I am working hard to share not only the good, but also the bad, and to ask God to help me react with my heart and not my emotions. I am a passionate person and it is easy for me to jump to conclusions. I am learning from my talks with God to pray first and react second.

God and I talk a lot on my walks. Christ Walk was intended to be a mind, body, and spiritual program. Being a very visual person, I find it inspiring to imagine God with me on my walks as though there is a real physical person along with me. I have wonderful insights on these walks. My heart beats stronger when I return, cleared of angst and worry and ready to take on the next challenge. My talk with God will usually provide me with an insight that I feel needs to be shared. For example, I share with God on these walks how very unqualified I feel to write this book. I fear the repercussions of sharing my faith and beliefs; I fear alienating some on their journey; I fear sharing the wrong thing or being misguided at this point in my life; I fear the call to proselytize; I fear that I am pontificating; I fear that I am not fit enough, thin enough, fast enough, good enough to write this. However, the call for Christ Walk is strong in my life and every time I have tried to put it aside, the call for it comes louder and stronger. Each time I have done Christ Walk, I am reminded that someone has been touched by it. No matter how weak I am in spirit, God will guide me through those moments. Each time I Christ Walk, God calls me to live this life again and share it to the best of my abilities. And that is all we can really do. The best of our abilities and the first fruits of our labor are for God; everything else is the gift of God's grace in our lives.

I want a healthy life and body and I know that no matter how many miles I walk, I can't do it on my own. I WANT God to be there every step of the way. I do not think that any miles walked to keep a healthy body will matter if God is not there first sharing the journey. There isn't much purpose to this temple if God is not a part of it, guiding me in what to do and how to do it. And because I am human there is often a battle going on between my will and God's will. Through prayer I can tame my will and allow God's will to work through me. My life is an entire prayer to God. Without God, I am not sure of my purpose here on earth.

Throughout the Bible, the story of God's people is about their relationship with God and their conversation with God through prayer. God hears all prayers and supplications:

Then hear in heaven their prayer and their plea, and maintain their cause.
—1 Kings 8:45b

If you search for "prayer" in a Bible search engine you will get thousands of verses of the prayers by various people and their relationships with God. Perhaps starting with the prayers of others will help you develop your discipline of prayer for yourself and your relationship with God. Sometimes we need to see how others had a relationship with God before we know how to move forward on our own. For some people, their relationship with God is innate; for others, it is a journey of faith in which they struggle. But whether day or night, good or bad, in tears or in joy, God IS with you in prayer.

By day the LORD *commands his steadfast love, and at night his song is with me, a prayer to the God of my life.* —Psalm 42:8

But know this, prayer is essential to your healthy life. It builds the temple just as surely as physical exercise and healthy eating.

God, be in my mind, God be in my heart, God be in my words that all of me is for you and with you and in you. Amen.

THOUGHTS TO PONDER

1. What is my prayer life like?

2. Do I feel more comfortable with intentional prayers or random conversations with God?

3. What sort of prayer discipline do I need to develop? What am I in search of during prayer time?

Therefore let all who are faithful offer prayer to you; at a time of distress, the rush of mighty waters shall not reach them. —Psalm 32:6

DAY 23   Steps taken: _____   Miles journeyed: _____

Exercise chosen: _____

Spiritual thoughts: _____

_____

_____

_____

_____

Feelings: _____

_____

_____

_____

_____

24 My Body Broken

BIBLICAL BIG IDEA # 24

Be gracious to me, O Lord, for I am languishing; O Lord,
heal me, for my bones are shaking with terror. —Psalm 6:2

The hardest challenge I have had to accept is the limitations of my body. Did I not just write several days ago that your limitations are usually built in your own mind and if you just plug away with it, that you will get there? With faith in God, you will get there? Well, that is true and I do believe that. I also believe there is a time and a place for everything. I also believe that everybody is different and capable of different things.

Since I was little, my body has challenged me. I was diagnosed as an asthmatic at the age of two and then had my autoimmune hearing loss at the age of twelve. Both of these, and the side effects of the medicine from my hearing loss, put a real crimp on some of my physical capabilities. When I took up running, I realized my stomach was sensitive to long distance running and had numerous complications when running long distances. The older I get the more and more impact I feel in my joints; a doctor has already told me that I have arthritis.

It is enough to make me want to roll over and not get out of bed some days. I am sure that people with cancer, diabetes, heart disease, and other illnesses feel the same way. There is nothing more frustrating than a body that will not do what you tell it to do, leaving you feeling completely at the mercy of what it will allow you to do. Again, I want to stress that there is a time and a place for everything. If you are going through an illness, or trying to figure out how to deal with a chronic diagnosis, give yourself time to figure out how to work with your body. On the one hand, the physical exercise and healthy eating can only help the management of your diagnosis. On the other hand, it *is* an illness and does affect how your body is going to respond on a day-to-day basis to physical exercise. If you are learning to manage a chronic illness for the first time, this may not be the best time to try to run your first marathon. You first need to learn to listen to your body. Then you can test its ability to take on new exercises and then just keep working at it. Never give up on seeing where you can go physically, even if you have a physical limitation.

So why does this happen? If I have the will, the joy, the power, the belief, and the conviction to take on a challenge, and I have faith that God will see me through it, why do I stumble? Why does my broken body defeat me? Why do people who have done everything "right" in their lives find themselves stricken with devastating illnesses or losses that threaten to cripple the very good person that they are? Why does each way I turn seem to have a bump in the road no matter what I do?

A dear friend of mine calls this the "human condition." For some reason, summing it up as the human condition feels like a cop out to me, but I have not come up with a better description. Perhaps the way my body reacts is not necessarily because of the choices that I have made, but it could be the choices that were made long ago in my genetic history that are affecting how my body reacts to the environment. The human body is adapting and evolving in order to learn how best to survive within the environment that we, as humans, have created. Some of the decisions in the world are made with every expectation of the greater good, but we have no knowledge of the impact of these decisions over lifetimes.

I am hesitant to make sweeping statements about the goodness or badness of inventions and changes in society. Often new inventions can improve the world in which we live. However, the span of our lives is short and the long-term implications of world changes are often unknown. Remember when the egg was vilified as bad and terrible for you? How cholesterol was the number-one killer? And overnight, the egg market was devastated, chickens grew horns, and all of a sudden, every American was looking for ways to reduce their cholesterol.

We have since learned that there are different kinds of cholesterols and fats and that not all are bad. In fact, our own body creates cholesterol. In the absence of taking in adequate cholesterol, our body makes MORE cholesterol. And that egg? The egg is a great source of protein, a good balance of nutrition with fats and cholesterol. Eggs are a power food! Now if you ate twelve eggs in a day—you might have problems. If you ate twelve bags of carrots in a day, you would have problems. The same can be said for avocados, coconuts, potatoes, and many other foods. I definitely look askance at sweeping statements about the negative or positive aspects of food and how bad or good they are for you, especially when they are food from God's earth. However, I also know that opium, marijuana, and tobacco are fruits of the earth and can be damaging. It is not the things themselves that are bad, it is what we do with them, how addictive they are, and how we as flawed humans handle that addiction.

Our fear of disease, death, and dying has prompted strides in science that have provided a means for addressing illness and disease. Unfortunately, the medical model also tends to encourage a "quick fix" approach to health management. We have been conditioned to look for the first pill we can pop to address our health concerns. We rarely give our bodies a chance to try to respond to imbalance, illness, and infection before we begin searching for that quick fix. We tend not to listen to our bodies when they are telling us to slow down and change pace, which often leads to injury and illness itself. We are too busy being busy to learn to listen to our bodies. Some of these illnesses and diseases we do bring upon ourselves—knowingly or unknowingly. I think some of the judgment of the world and our actions are played out in our body.

This is not to say that illness and disease are judgments from God. I do not believe that God subjects us to illness as punishment. However, I do think with the freedom of choice that God gives us that illnesses and disease are often the results of choices (by ourselves or others) that impact our own individual lives. My father's choice to continue to smoke probably contributed to my asthma as a child and his stroke as an adult. Do I blame my father? Not really; it would be a really pointless endeavor to do so, and who knows what log I have in my own eye in the choices I make about my health. However, people want to seek the "why" of illnesses and injury, death, and disease and we have to come to realize that all of these things are a part of the human condition. There will NEVER be a time when illness, disease, and injury do not occur. There will NEVER be a time when we don't all die (in the physical sense). This is the nature of our human existence.

Disease and illness can open many individuals to a greater relationship with God. Individuals that seek the "why" of their illnesses move from the unfulfilling answers of the human dimension to the answers in the spiritual dimension where they find solace, healing, and peace. No drug can provide the comfort and healing of spiritual succour. God's loving kindness is there with us through any trial and tribulation of the human body; loving kindness will transcend whatever broken body you may be challenged with.

Judgment is the result of all choices made. Judgment is what we do to ourselves (individually and collectively) with the freedom that God gave us. Judgment is also how we deal with all the consequences that are either self-inflicted, or inflicted by actions beyond our control. Judgment is the choice to be in communion with God through it all, or to turn your back with blame, reviling God as the source of evil and pain in your life. Surely God can take your anger and pain—God has taken much of my own. I have not turned my back on God during my struggles and afflictions, and I hope I never will.

THOUGHTS TO PONDER

1. Do you struggle with your body? Do you feel your body is broken?

2. Do you feel your health is your judgment for your life?

3. How can you come to reconciliation and move past this stage of judgment?

For all of us must appear before the judgment seat of Christ, so that each may receive recompense for what has been done in the body, whether good or evil.
—2 Corinthians 5:10

DAY 24   Steps taken: _____   Miles journeyed: _____

Exercise chosen: _____

Spiritual thoughts: _____

_____

_____

_____

Feelings: _____

_____

_____

_____

DAY 25 Your Journey Backpack

BIBLICAL BIG IDEA #25

His divine power has given us everything needed for life and godliness, through the knowledge of him who called us by his own glory and goodness. —2 Peter 1:3

Every journey has a backpack. Every lifetime fills a backpack with the tools, tricks, and successes to get through all the journeys of a lifetime. If Christ is in your backpack, all the skills and tools will fall into place when you need them. Practicing a Christ-centered lifestyle makes picking the right tools and the right choices at each stage of your journey easier.

Life is a series of crossroads. Some roads may be more visibly wrong than others. At some crossroads you may pitch a tent for many months before deciding on a direction. Some roads are not necessarily better than other roads. At some crossroads, it matters more what we do once we are on these journeys; it is a matter of choice. All of life is a matter of choice because God gave us that freedom. In your backpack should be a Bible. No matter how confusing or contradictory the Bible may seem to be, through diligence in study, it is the ONLY document we have of God's relationship with God's people. Studying with the Bible can help you through your conflicts and discern how God's word speaks to you. I have been through enough Bible studies to realize that the Bible says a lot of different things to different people in different ways and at different points in their lives. I have found that once where I saw conflict and discord within stories, it was due to a point in my life influencing my thoughts rather than the true context of events. Perception colors the Bible, perception colors your journey, and, well, perception really colors everything.

Your perception of events will be colored by your attitude. If your perception of events colors your understanding, then your attitude is also going to influence your perception. If you perceive an event to be challenging, frustrating, or debilitating, a good attitude can offset your perception of an event to make it a positive experience. Likewise, if you have a negative attitude and a negative perception of an event, your experience of the event will be perceived as negative.

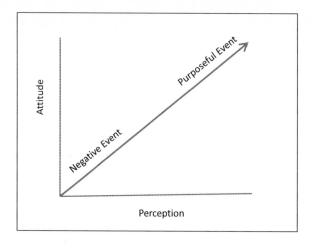

Given our freedom and God's love, we choose our perception and attitude. Whether we are trying to live a healthier life, lose weight, get more fit, take control of our health, relationships, interactions with others, stress, job, addictions, or spirituality, there is nothing that others "do" for us, nor can we change what others do. Rather, we can work on our perception of and attitude toward an event and take control of what we as individuals can control, letting go of those things that are outside those boundaries. When I perceive myself to be lacking choices or lacking control over the situation, I find that my attitude tends to spiral down. When I am able to reexamine my perception of an event, pray about it, and come to peace with it, my attitude greatly improves.

When I was losing my hearing, I had a variety of different perceptions as I worked through my grief of losing this sense. I sat in church so incredibly angry at God that I felt (and perceived) that I could not participate in the worship because I could not hear. I could not hear the music, the sermon, the joyous prayers of the Eucharist and I felt terribly, terribly sad, frustrated, mad, abandoned, and angry during the experience. And my heartfelt cry of anguish was heard by God. And God said to me, "It does not matter if you can or cannot hear." My perception of the church service and my experience of the liturgy shifted. I did not need to hear to experience God's love and I did not NEED to hear to have a purpose in life. It has transformed how I experience my life and my relationships. I have a purpose no matter what.

Several years after the experience, I was trying to articulate how I felt about that perfect moment of communion with God. It was unlike any experience I have ever had in my life. I wrote the following with a nod to John Milton:

On Deafness

Deafness means to be without sound
And yet I seem to hear
A noise that levels mountains
And calms the frightened deer
A song that sings without voices
A Beethoven-like symphony
That echoes, echoes, echoes, in my quiet ear
A loss that I felt for such a small while
Was soon lost in a beauty I was now to see
A soundless life-vibrance, a hearing person would never presume
They think that I miss out, and sometimes I do
But a loss that brought a gift so fair
Makes my deafness hard to rue
When a different sound came to me
That never before I knew.
(1995)

My perception and attitude of the events in my life radically changed because God called me, and everything I needed in my toolbox started there. Since then my toolbox has grown to include the Bible, my perceptions and attitude, knowledgeable professionals, friends, and relationships, perseverance, priorities, and faith. With faith, anything is possible. With faith, my spirit is healthy and growing.

From a physical perspective, I have found that setting priorities in my life is very important. I have priorities for prayer, worship, family, study, and physical exercise. It is not self-indulgent for me to consider my physical exercise and healthy eating a priority because I feel very strongly it is important for me to take care of my body and keep it strong so that I can be there for my family, my friends, my church, and my work. My strong body will get me through the things I am called to do. As a result, my priorities and beliefs have become a part of my toolbox in dealing with life events as they are thrown at me.

Several days ago I wrote about risk factors. I have an insane number of risk factors in my genetic makeup: stroke, diabetes, heart disease, cancer, and depression. There is nothing that tends to invoke fear in me more than the thought of not doing everything I can to offset the risk of being in a nursing home as I age. I have jokingly said that I would ideally like to go as hard and strong and as fast as I can until I can go no longer, but I have no desire to linger on in a bed unable to do those things. Now that might still happen, and I know God will be with me should that come to pass, but in the meantime, God has given me the strength and skills to counteract some of those risk factors. It is important to me that my health is a part of the priorities I have set.

Does any of this mean that my perception and attitude do not falter? It happens all the time. *I reset my perception and attitude through prayer.* My friends and family help me put my attitude back in perspective when it is challenged. I know that when my attitude and perspective deteriorates, it usually means I have not been opening my heart to God to have those talks that put me back where I need to be. If you are having a hard time with perception and attitude, there are people there to help. If you are feeling a gaping hole (or wall, or river—however you visualize it) in your spirit, your priest or pastor can help you work on connecting to your God-spark so that it feels lit within you. It is there. I know it, I believe it, and I bet others can see it far more easily than you can see it in yourself. Just like a candle needs oxygen to burn, you need to fan the flames of your God-spark with prayer and meditation and relationships. The more you open yourself to love and share love, the more you feel Christ in your life. And the more you have Christ in your life, the bigger your toolbox of skills and talents gets to help you through any of the crossroads you meet on your journey.

THOUGHTS TO PONDER

1. What is in my current toolbox, backpack, or pocketbook that I will carry on my journey?

2. What is missing and how can I find it?

3. Where do you think your perception and attitude fall on the continuum?

For a holy and disciplined spirit will flee from deceit,
and will leave foolish thoughts behind,
and will be ashamed at the approach of unrighteousness.

For wisdom is a kindly spirit,
but will not free blasphemers from the guilt of their words;
because God is witness of their inmost feelings,
and a true observer of their hearts, and a hearer of their tongues.
—The Wisdom of Solomon 1:5–7

DAY 25 Steps taken: _____ Miles journeyed: _____

Exercise chosen: _____

Spiritual thoughts: _____

_____

_____

_____

_____

Feelings: _____

_____

_____

_____

_____

Family Time

BIBLICAL BIG IDEA #26

So let us not grow weary in doing what is right, for we will reap at harvest time, if we do not give up. So then, whenever we have an opportunity, let us work for the good of all, and especially for those of the family of faith. —Galatians 6:9–10

In the tradition of the ancient church, children were baptized as infants alongside the head of household as a sign that this was a family of God. Baptism continued as families and individuals grew together in the spirit of Christ and created their communities of God. When baptism occurs, it is not only building the family of the church, but it is building a family of faith that starts at home. If you come from a tradition that baptizes later in life, this is also amazing. Actually, I think *any* baptism is amazing. I am awed when children and adults step forth to take on their own baptism, showing they are committing to their family of faith on their own two feet. I think baptism at any point on the continuum of life is a good thing. Every step we make to build the family of faith is right.

Faith starts in the home. Before there were churches and temples, there were rites in the home that signified a holy family or a family of God. The blessing of food and breaking of bread together in the home were early versions of the Christian rite of Holy Communion. Sharing of Bible stories in the home was the first organized Bible study. We pass on the teachings of Christ to future generations when we share God's story at home. The teachings of Jesus and the church began and developed from the home before they ever reached the structure of a physical church building. As my family prays together, we are bringing God into our home. My father used to tell me that "Families that pray together, stay together."

"For where two or three are gathered in my name, I am there among them."
—Matthew 18:20

I pray each night that God helps me to raise and grow a good Christian family. I want my children to know God and experience God as my husband and I have. I want them to have that RELATIONSHIP that transcends all relationships and I constantly worry that, although I have brought them to the trough, they will not drink. My fear that my children will not know God is one fear I must give to God. I know that my children will be raised in the church and experience God through rites and worship, but it is only through God that they will find that relationship. I cannot make that for them. I question how well I bring them up in a family of faith, and pray that over time my children's relationship with God will blossom. Right now, my nine-year-old son's view of God is very concrete, and he is struggling to place it in the context of his life. Recently, he peppered my husband with questions. "Did space create the big bang, or did the big bang create space?" "Did God create the big bang, or did the big bang create God?" "If God created the big bang, where was he before that?" On the one hand, I am thrilled that he is asking these questions, but on the other hand, I worry that my little scientist will rationalize God into a box. Both my husband and I are devoted to bringing up our children in this family of faith and continuing to pray together through all of the crazy questions and hope that one day our son will find his own path to God.

Family time is one of my priorities along with a healthy, Christ-centered life. It is natural to me that the activities of my life revolve around what our family does with church and what our family does in physical activities. I enjoy spending time with my children enjoying God in nature and experiencing everything given to us in this world. We are avid travellers, hikers, and bikers. We take our kids with us on most occasions and challenge them to hike as far as they can hike and explore what may be beyond the next hill. For the most part my seven-year-old daughter likes to experience these times together from my husband's shoulders. I think she likes the view and she can whisper sweet chatter at her daddy whom she adores. My son and I take off together. We have learned to pack little "energy pills" of M&Ms in our pockets for when the children's energy flags. I have never been more proud of my son than when, at the age of five, he hiked to Panorama Point on Mount Rainier under his own steam, even though the park ranger said it was too difficult for a kid his age. This was not a hike for the faint of heart, let alone a five-year-old, but he had the right attitude and the right perseverance that day to be successful. That day we enjoyed glorious exercise, in God's glorious creation, with our family, and we talked about how God made the world. It was one of those days when all of my priorities fell in place and all was well with the world.

We have also begun teaching our kids about giving and tithing. The concept of money is growing for my kids and we are trying to teach them that the first fruits of our labor need to go to God. We are teaching them to give, save, and spend—but spending should only happen once we have given first to God and those in need. It is challenging to teach young children to think of others first when they are so inclined to think of themselves first. This is natural. As children grow and become aware, they are consumed with how their bodies feel, what they can do, where they came from. Children are all about themselves at this stage of their lives. They first explore the world of their family. Then, their concern grows for extended family and friends. As their love of family grows, they are then able to develop compassion for others. Some adults are learning this, too. I believe that we need to first feel love in a safe environment before our compassion for others develops.

Our churches become another very important family for teaching this compassion. We are brought up in a society that reinforces that life is about me, me, me and you, you, you and not necessarily about *us* as a community. We need the love in churches and families to teach that we, as a collective group, make the world a better place together for others.

Just like children, adults have difficulty learning that when they give the fruits of the labor and money to God first, then the rest of their priorities will fall together. How many people do you know who despite all their worldly success are miserable people because money and fame bring empty satisfaction? It is when those individuals learn to use their wealth and fame for others first that they begin to derive satisfaction from their purpose.

This time with my family (whether it is part of a healthy life and activities, exploring God's great creations, teaching about tithing, compassion, money, others, or worship) is part of our Christian calling as parents. Through these activities, we are building the bride of Christ—the church. The church is a family we build together. Through the communion of believers we are given the opportunity to share our experiences with God and develop the body of knowledge about the relationship of God with God's people. It is our collective experience that begins to tell the story of this amazing relationship throughout time, and this starts first in the home.

My husband and I did not have children for many years. For a number of years I think I was too selfish to have kids. I had not gotten it out of my system that my life would no longer be controlled by me, but rather by the forces of nature that are my children. In a way, I am truly thankful that it took a long time to have children, because even though I have small kids and have had a number of years with them now, I am constantly taken aback by how hard it is to be a parent. I thought that as long as I brought my children up in a loving, disciplined home and molded them with good behavior, kindness, church, and a healthy environment, that all would be well. I failed to take into consideration their individual personalities! And how lovely and amazing those personalities are! However, they come with their own wants, desires, and needs, and I am constantly reminded that, for now, while I have these two under my care, I am ultimately responsible for them. My time is not my own. I have had to learn that there is a time and place for everything under heaven, but at this time in my life, my calling, my *vocare*, my mission as a part of God's church is to raise these children.

If and when you decided (or will decide) to have children, you took on an additional discipline of crafting new members of God's world and raising them to love one another. The first step in raising them is to love your children unconditionally and show them what God's love is like. We do this by making family our priority and putting aside our individual pursuits for the short time we have our children. The best advice and gift I get regularly from my friends and family is not to rush these years with the children. They will be gone soon enough. No matter how bad or difficult they may be, it is a phase. Continue with loving discipline and ensure they know that they are a priority in your life. This is your time to teach them about a healthy mind, body, and spirit. You are responsible for weaving healthy habits, a healthy spirituality, and healthy minds as a part of how they will become adults. When children are nurtured, loved, and kept safe, they will know that they live in a family of faith, too.

THOUGHTS TO PONDER

1. How do I feel about family time?

2. Do I make enough family time, or do I tend to want to spend time in my own pursuits? How can I make more family time and make it enjoyable for all?

3. How do I feel about my family of faith?

So then, whenever we have an opportunity, let us work for the good of all, and especially for those of the family of faith. —Galatians 6:10

DAY 26   Steps taken: _____   Miles journeyed: _____

Exercise chosen: _____

Spiritual thoughts: _____

_____

_____

_____

_____

Feelings: _____

_____

_____

_____

_____

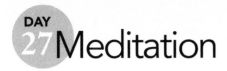

Meditation

BIBLICAL BIG IDEA #27

Live by the Spirit, I say, and do not gratify the desires of the flesh. —Galatians 5:16

Meditation is a mental discipline that targets clearing and quieting the mind in order to find inner peace. Or in my mind, "Hush up Anna and *listen!*" Meditation practices can be found in most any religious as well as many secular disciplines. From a Christian perspective, meditation is a form of prayer in which we use breathing techniques and spiritual words to quiet and clear the mind in order to hear the Holy Spirit. There are many ways to achieve a meditative state. Some people use certain prayers, breathing, gongs, chants, bells, or guided methods to reach this state of meditation. Meditation does not have to take long. Research indicates that as little as ten to fifteen minutes of meditation a day can produce enormous benefits for the body. I use a form of meditative walking in order to clear my mind and focus on God.

Walking is one of my most spiritual activities. During my walk, I am able to set a rhythm that allows me to clear my mind and focus on God. Initially my walk is pavement pounding as I am usually releasing stress, anxiety, and frustration from my day. Then, as I clear my thoughts and emotions, I am able to set a rhythm that smoothes out and develops a cadence in time with my breath. I breathe in from my nose with one step and exhale on another. I find that this pattern allows me to settle my spirit and hear God on my walks. I often use a repetitious phrase, such as "Yahweh" or "Jesus, Lamb of God, have mercy upon us" as I begin this cycle of my walk. Sometimes I simply say, "Here I am Lord," and open my spirit to be with God. The motion of walking helps me to still my busy mind so that I pray and listen more effectively to God. There is also the added bonus that it is good for me! The purpose of meditation is to be silent: to still your mind, slow your breathing, and allow God to speak to you in the silence of your soul. I am able to do this through walking. I call this meditative walking. You may prefer to meditate at rest in a soothing place that you have called your own.

Either way, meditation is very good for the body. As a type of prayer, it is a discipline that draws us closer to God. As a discipline of health, it lowers our resting heart rate, decreases blood pressure, releases the good hormones, and reduces the release of stress hormones. Meditation is an excellent discipline that helps to control cravings, addictions, mood swings, frustrations, stress, and all sorts of health concerns. Meditation is a cornerstone of a healthy life that is often overlooked. I do not know about you, but I am often overwhelmed by what I *have* to do to be healthy: watch what I eat, exercise at least an hour a day, meditate, pray, etc. etc. etc. The list goes on and on. God never said it was easy being human. I find that my meditative walk allows me to prioritize those things that I have to do and manage that list so that it does not overwhelm me. My walk (or whatever exercise I choose for the day) tends to put things in perspective so that I can handle the challenges of the remainder of the day with aplomb.

I have often been accused of being an excessive worrier. I come from a long line of worriers. I have been told that if I am worrying so much, I am not really trusting God to take care of my worries. If you are a worrier like me, then your answer was probably similar to mine—if I am not worrying (and I honestly do not think of it as worrying, but more like thinking about things a lot), then nothing would get done. My thoughts and thinking help me work through the concerns on my mind so that I can talk to God about them and then move on. I am a doer. What people may fail to realize about me (and you, if you are like me) is that my worries are there, they are a part of who I am, but I am able to deal with them by sharing my worries with God through my prayer and meditative walking. When I am not sharing these worries with God, they tend to overwhelm me and then nothing gets done. This is one of the primary reasons I walk and I talk with God while I walk. Not only does it help me to deal with my worry list, but it puts them in perspective so that I can deal with them. Worrying is not necessarily a bad thing when you have a constructive way to deal with it.

Another benefit of meditative walking is that it distracts you from the urge for food, smoking, drugs, caffeine, stress, and anxiety. When you walk with the Spirit, your body feels gratified by what you are doing and who you are with, not what you think your body wants and desires. When you think about walking with God, you start to think about how you are going to walk *for* God in your day-to-day life. You begin to think about taking these steps from being about you and your health to using the strength you gain from this healthy activity to make others healthy. I have mentioned before that my running was never enjoyable when it was about me. When taking care of myself became less about me, and more about being strong and fit to take care of my family and others, then I was empowered to do something good for myself. It was not a selfish or self-centered endeavor.

Meditative walking differs from other types of exercise, as it is not necessarily focused on time, distance, intensity, or other measurable goals. Meditative walking is using the rhythm of walking and breathing to open yourself to the Word of God. It is a great time to pray, but it is also a great time to listen. A lot of people spend a great deal of their time in prayer talking to God—which is good, don't get me wrong—but then we spend a lot less time listening to God and hearing what God's goal for us in this world will be.

I am also a victim of this fault. I talk a lot. I have to stop myself so that I take the time to listen. We chatter on about forgiveness, guidance, help, praise, thanksgiving, blessings, and repentance, but often we stop the prayer there and do not take the time to hear God's forgiveness, guidance, reprimand, or direction. We feel good knowing that Jesus made the ultimate sacrifice for our sins. We know that God will love us anyway, and we feel good that we have gotten our burdens off our shoulders and onto God's, but then, what? Do we stop and listen? Do we take a moment to be filled with the Holy Spirit so that we can be moved to better behavior, stronger convictions, or clear direction? I find I am often too busy talking and not quiet enough to listen in my relationship with God. The noise of the world is very distracting from the sounds of heaven.

While you are challenging yourself in this forty-day walking program to take yourself a little farther and a little longer each day with your walk with Christ, I encourage you to try meditative walking. You will need to practice the smooth heel-to-toe walking and consistent breathing so that your mind will quiet. Come up with a phrase that helps you get to this place and repeat it. Or download some spiritual chants and music onto your music player and clear your mind to hear God's word. God speaks to me loud and clear on many of my walks, I am sure that God will talk to you as well if you take the time to listen.

My prayer for you in Christ Walk is this:

Christ Walk Prayer

I will try this day to walk the path set before me
I will try to walk a little longer, a little stronger
I will walk with my mind, body, and spirit
I will walk with others, I will walk for others
I will walk when others cannot
I will be still and know that you are God on the days I cannot walk

I will walk with you Lord, on the path you set before me
When my own feet fail, I know you will help me get up and
    walk again
I will imagine what it would be like to walk in Christ's shoes
And try to live my life as though I was on Christ's path
I will pray that I walk the path I am called to and not turn down paths
I am not
Today, Lord, on my journey I will Christ Walk
And I am thankful that you Christ Walk with me too.
Amen.

THOUGHTS TO PONDER

1. What do you think about meditative walking? Have you tried it?

2. What was your experience with meditative walking? What did you
hear from God?

3. Are you a worrier like me? Does meditative walking help you with
your worries? Do you control your worries and give them to God, or
do they control you?

*Therefore I tell you, do not worry about your life, what you will eat or what you
will drink, or about your body, what you will wear. Is not life more than food,
and the body more than clothing? Look at the birds of the air; they neither sow
nor reap nor gather into barns, and yet your heavenly Father feeds them. Are
you not of more value than they? And can any of you by worrying add a single
hour to your span of life?* —Matthew 6:25–27

DAY 27   Steps taken: _____   Miles journeyed: _____

Exercise chosen: _____

Spiritual thoughts: _____

_____

_____

Feelings: _____

_____

_____

DAY
28 Making Smart, Small Changes

BIBLICAL BIG IDEA #28

Then the spirit of the LORD will possess you, and you will be in a prophetic frenzy along with them and be turned into a different person. —1 Samuel 10:6

It is very difficult to write a book intended for people with a variety of fitness levels and make it valuable for changing yourself not just physically, but also mentally and spiritually. We are all made differently. Those differences give us different challenges to overcome when we start a spiritual endeavor. No matter whether you seek to run the fastest or farthest you have ever gone, or have selected the longest distance in the Bible during your Christ Walk journey, or if you are getting off the couch for the first time in twenty years, these decisions and changes are all made successfully with smart, small changes. Just thinking about taking on this challenge is the first step in the right direction. The next step is to make one change at a time and then keep making those changes until you are changing your entire lifestyle.

If the couch potato decides to run a marathon, then the individual will set themselves up for frustration, injury, and potential failure. Making change occurs in increments. Just like salvation—you first accept God into your heart, and then the change in you evolves over a lifetime. Your journey as a Christian begins with baptism in the Christian covenant. I do not believe it ends there. When you have been called to be a Christian, you then begin making decisions about your life based on Christian beliefs: to first love one another.

With change in our physical selves, we need to make the decision to exercise more, be healthier, and pray more often. This is a part of developing our bodies towards Christ's call in our life. Then each day, small choices and changes can be made to be healthier.

If you want to improve your physical exercise—set a goal. For Christ Walk, you have probably chosen to walk a certain distance based on one of many biblical routes. The next time you do Christ Walk, I challenge you to choose a harder and longer route. For some individuals, you will set a goal of five miles every day during the challenge; for others, you may start with a mile and work yourself up to four or five miles, depending on the challenge. If you really want to run a marathon, set your first goal to train for a 5K, then a 10K, then a half marathon, and then a full marathon. Consider dedicating your goal to raise money for a mission or something you believe in. This combines your physical pursuits with your spiritual calling.

This is a *lifetime* of challenges. This is a *lifetime* of promises dedicating your body and your health to do Christ's work in the world. Just because you may complete one goal, it does not mean there are not other goals around the corner. Just because we have built a school for children without education, does not mean there is not another community that needs our love and concern just as much. The call for Christ's acts in the world does not end with one good deed. We are called to keep our bodies strong for what we are called to do in our lives.

For athletes, once they have attained their goal of completing a marathon, a triathlon, or a bike race, they then look at their time and consider, "How can I go faster?" or "Is there a longer challenge?" or perhaps "Is there something new I have yet to try?" Athletes constantly look at ways to improve themselves—this is why Christ Walk can work for anyone. There are many routes in the Bible for many different fitness levels. The question is, how will you take it to the next level? And then, how will you maintain the health level that you have gained?

Another way of looking at change is to use the FIT principle. The FIT principle stands for Frequency, Intensity, and Time. The key to the FIT principle is to change two of the three fitness areas when adjusting your exercise so that you are ensuring a safe and healthy challenge and change to your routine. Research shows that if you try to change all three components of FIT, you are more likely to induce injury, illness, and fatigue and put yourself further back than where you started. For example, when I was learning to increase my miles for my half marathon, I started by increasing the frequency of my runs. I began with running two days per week, and worked up to running four days per week. On my fourth run, I focused on increasing time or distance (distance can equate to intensity, but can also be increased by increasing speed). Each time I ran a little farther (I would increase my distance runs by 10% of the previous distance). I trained my body to tolerate more and more effort. Over a twelve-week period, I worked my way up to fourteen miles thereby ensuring I could do the 13.1 required by the half marathon. I did not get sick, injured, or excessively fatigued during my training time. I was successfully able to complete my goal and have since run two half marathons and a ten-miler. My new goals are related to strength training and power lifting. I am using the same principles to mix up my routine and ensure my body is a healthy, fit machine to do God's work.

Intensity is how hard you are pushing your body. It can be scientifically calculated at what percentage of your maximum heart rate that you are working. As you work in your target heart zone, you are training your heart (strengthening the heart muscle) to adapt to hard levels of exercise. This makes the heart respond, pumping more efficiently to the body and the muscles that are performing work. Once upon a time, our bodies naturally adapted to the physical activity associated with the work we did. As we trained to learn a craft or skilled labor, our bodies naturally built up the stamina and strength to do this work. Now that our work is centered on computers and other non-mobile work, our bodies have to be re-taught this skill. This is why we exercise. Our bodies were always meant to move. When we do not use the muscles in the temple God has given us, they get flabby and atrophied. It takes more and more training to get them to work again. No one said it was easy! But just like your body, or prayer, or learning a new skill, if we do not use it, we lose it.

You also can use all of these principles for any sport or activity. If you are a first-time walker, then you will use these same principles for increasing your mileage and taking your walk to the next level. Do not think you have to run a half or full marathon. You can walk it, if that is your goal. Or be content to finally get off the couch and enjoy your environment. Only you can determine the health level you seek. Perhaps your goals will be focusing on increasing your exercise and improving your diet just enough to get off of diabetes or high blood pressure medications—these are both fantastic goals. What do you want? What will make your body stronger to support your calling? Will you be able to play with your children or grandchildren more? Chase them? Play sports with them? Will you be able to build a house for a mission team? Whatever your goals, this is an opportunity to make your body stronger to do whatever it is that you have dreamed about doing for God.

If you wish you improve your eating habits, you first have to look at where you are eating poorly, and this means keeping a food journal. As painful as it sounds, it really is important to record everything you eat. We constantly underestimate the amount we eat and overestimate the amount we work out. Diets fail when we make massive changes to our eating patterns. The body thinks we are depriving it of what it wants and it releases stress hormones, which make us feel hungrier and less satisfied when we have made such a drastic change. I have tried a variety of diets—high-protein, carb-free, the cabbage soup diet, the blood-type diet, and others at various points in my life. I finally wised up and realized that I like food too much to make anything forbidden. I also like a great deal of variety. The only two ways I have ever been successful in losing weight were following Weight Watchers and cutting out processed food (i.e., eating real food in moderation). Both allowed me a wide variety of choices, nothing was forbidden, and each made me consciously make decisions about the food I placed in my mouth and the tradeoffs I would choose to make if I want to indulge.

I have always been fit and active. However, following the birth of my second child, I somehow ended up at 234 pounds. To this day, I am not sure how I let that happen. I was shocked, depressed, disappointed, and completely frustrated at how difficult it was to get the weight to go. I exercised through both pregnancies. I thought I was eating healthy, but I guess I did not, since I quit writing it all down and was not consciously making decisions. Unfortunately, I have the type of metabolism that if I choose to have a cupcake now, then my trade off will have to be to walk a little longer, have a salad at dinner, or forego a glass of wine. I am also honest enough to admit that I would rather exercise a little more to have more flexibility in my diet than deny myself foods I like. I had to find the line where I was comfortable with my tradeoffs. For example, I cannot go without cream in my coffee and I think the fat-free stuff tastes like plastic. I can, however, measure out two teaspoons versus two tablespoons and still be satisfied. I draw the line at diet food. Diet food is processed food, engineered food. I have already said God gave us everything we need on the earth to be healthy and have wonderful food, so I would rather savour a small bit of real dark chocolate than have an entire diet chocolate bar. God did not grow meal replacement bars on trees in the Garden of Eden.

Over the years, as I have made these small, conscious decisions, I have found that my pantry is not as full as it used to be. I stock a lot less packaged food, and would rather fill my refrigerator with fresh options. I have recently bought into a Cooperative Shared Agriculture (CSA) program, what I call my "farm box," and have been delighted to try new things, experiment, and develop a relationship with my farming group by sharing recipes and experiences from what I discover in my box. The added benefit is that I am getting produce at the peak of the season and eating in sync with the growing season, rather than the greenhouse one. I am supporting local farmers, supporting practices that are better for the environment, and doing something that is great for my family. I have also been making a lot of changes towards organic produce and as much raw material as I can find. I have rediscovered cooking and my love of it. I choose to snack on nuts versus chips when I want crunch, and if I am going to have ice cream, it will be the real thing.

These changes did not happen overnight and I am sure there will be fluctuation in it over time. But I started with one thing and then as I felt better and better, I made healthier choices. I know my body well enough now that I listen to it and nourish it with good meats, vegetables, and fruits. The more real food I eat (while paying attention to the amount) the healthier I am. I am also enough of a foodie that I have to write it down. I will cheat. Most of us will cheat because no one is holding our hand telling us not to.

If you want to improve your prayer life or mental and spiritual life, you will also need to make changes in your day-to-day structure to include that. Just as you carve out time to exercise, carve out time to pray, meditate, and listen. You do not have to do these things all on your own. Having a friend and/or family member committing to a healthy journey with you builds accountability. It also helps build relationships and love, which is precious to God.

I hope you have realized that none of these healthy changes are being driven by the desire to be thin or to be anything more than the beautiful gift God created. We are all made in God's image in various sizes or shapes. It has taken me a long time to realize that I can be healthy, but that a drive for eating and physical activity towards being skinny is really self-centered. Being skinny doesn't necessarily mean you are closer to God, or a better person, or healthier. In fact, there are a lot of skinny people who are probably very unhealthy. Making these changes is about building a stronger temple for God, to do God's work in the world. It is not about creating a new you to meet the ideal image you have crafted in your brain. If along the Christ Walk way, you lose weight, slim down, get stronger, faster, more toned—AWESOME—put that new body towards God's work. It's God's temple, not yours.

THOUGHTS TO PONDER

1. Take a look at your pantry—what can you get rid of? What can you replace it with that is healthy?

2. Can you walk longer, farther, stronger this week?

3. Can you make small changes to stop at one soda (or none at all), get rid of the empty food, take the stairs, ride your bike, park the car farther?

4. What will you do this week that is a little further on your Christ Walk?

Do you not know that in a race the runners all compete, but only one receives the prize? Run in such a way that you may win it. —1 Corinthians 9:24

DAY 28 Steps taken: _____ Miles journeyed: _____

Exercise chosen: _____

Spiritual thoughts: _____

_____

_____

_____

Feelings: _____

_____

_____

_____

PULSE CHECK REPENTANCE

What is repentance? Repentance is being fully engaged in the process of forgiveness with God. God's grace forgave us before we knew we needed forgiving. Jesus' sacrifice and crucifixion paid the ultimate "payment" for whatever ills our sins create. I believe that there is life after death. I believe in the communion of all the saints and the chorus of the heavenly host. I believe that our acts of repentance are those behaviors we learn to repeat over and over, trying to move ourselves from sinful actions to actions with grace. Through God's strength, I am able to create new behaviors that are healthy: mind, body, and spirit. Through God's grace, I can mess up multiple times and my prayers of repentance help me get up and try again to live gracefully. Because I am human, I will sin often. I am awed that no matter how many times I stray from graceful living, God's forgiveness allows me the chance to try again; to move away from actions that are harmful to my body and soul. Because I am engaged in an active relationship with God, my cycle of sin, forgiveness, and repentance is active. I believe that every positive goal I set is one that shows an act of repentance, allowing me to move closer to a life of righteousness. I believe that a life of health is one that is full of prayer, work, physical exercise, eating, sleep, and love. Because of my humanness, I will constantly be setting new goals of righteous living and behavior. I will also have to repent for those actions that are not. Through my perseverance and faith in God, my acts of repentance will lead me closer to a healthier life: body, mind, and soul.

The act of repentance is how I show that I am fully engaged with an active and healthy life with God. I am able to repent and try again because God loves me as I am, is fully engaged in my life, and redeems me through grace.

PART FIVE

REDEMPTION

A Chapter for Spouses
(My Tribute to
Military Spouses)

BIBLICAL BIG IDEA #29
*Therefore a man leaves his father and his mother and clings
to his wife, and they become one flesh.* —Genesis 2:24

My husband and I have had to be physically separated multiple times in our marriage due to work travel, deployments, and family illnesses. Whether the time apart is a couple of days, a week, or many months, we never are really happy. God joined us together when we got married, and I truly feel that part of me is missing when we are not together. I may jokingly talk about a "girls' weekend" or "I need to get away," but when I do have to be separated from my family, I usually pine for my husband and children. I do not think I can separate my family from who I am as an individual anymore. When we are apart, I miss them terribly. I feel I am missing a part of myself, as clichéd as it may sound.

As a military family, we have been lucky thus far in that my husband's deployments have been spaced at reasonable intervals. Nonetheless, when the Army calls, our spouses go. I find it very difficult to describe a deployment. As a spouse, I am incredibly proud of my soldier for the gift he gives our country. Every soldier takes an oath to uphold the Constitution and freedoms of the United States. Many soldiers feel called to their chosen profession and that they are helping to make the world a better place and create areas where others are allowed the same freedoms that we enjoy. Soldiers go to war with the belief they are working to make the world a better place. Most soldiers do not believe their mission is to sow discord and discontent. They are often freeing people from oppressive leadership. I have heard many anti-Christian remarks against the military over time, and while in my heart my prayers are for peace and love throughout the world, I also think it is a sin to look away from areas in the world where we can make a difference. I have struggled theologically to discern whether or not war is evil, or if war is the godly choice when there are people who are beaten down, trodden under the yoke of oppression, and unable to know God's love because of religious persecution. Many theologians have written on when war is justified.

Right, wrong or indifferent, I believe that in the United States our soldiers are called to war to defend our freedom, including the right to worship as we choose, and to help create a world where others have those same freedoms. I do not believe that dictators or terrorists are a part of God's vision for the world. Our soldiers help to defend our freedom and secure freedoms for others in order to make a world where people can worship as they are called to do.

A spouse at home has his or her own call to support his/her service member, raise children, pray, and work to a stronger self with God's help when the soldier is gone. I do not think that a military spouse's sacrifice is necessarily greater than another's sacrifice, but it is very different. It is difficult to explain how we must always be hopeful and vigilant with our prayers, and have faith that God will protect our spouses. God's strength and steadfastness is often the only strength that gets us through a deployment. I do not think I could be strong through a deployment without God there with me.

Along with prayer, devotion to physical exercise is often paramount to our sanity. I am awed by military spouses who look at these times as an opportunity to grow as an individual—to grow stronger in body, mind, and spirit because it is an event in our lives that is like no other. I have known the strength of military spouses to bloom during these trying times by training for their first marathon, or half marathon, or triathlon. They take on positions in non-profit organizations to raise money and items for children in the countries where their spouses are deployed. When their soldiers fall, they gather the shreds of their life and build a new one, creating running groups that are a living memory to the fallen soldiers across the land. There are families that create photographic testimonies to the sacrifice of these soldiers to ensure that no soldier's sacrifice is ever forgotten. These families that not only support their soldier as they deploy, but also when they die, are the strongest families I know. They are living testaments to a life in God in the midst of strife.

When God cleaved military families together, he equipped them with special skills to withstand the separation together. I know each time that my husband and I were separated, my goal was to come out stronger for myself, my kids, and my family. I knew that having a strong family at home made it so much easier for my spouse to do his job. And through

God's grace, we have survived these separations and will continue to survive them in the years to come.

Setting goals during trying times should be considered great therapy. Goals give us something else to think about during these times. These goals, just like Lenten goals, could be things such as walking, running, or racing goals. It could be to prayerfully read a book together with your spouse while you are separated. It could be to take on a new goal at church that you prayerfully stick with despite the trying times you are experiencing. Goals give us a sense of purpose. Purpose provides a call through trying times. God's grace lends us strength and power to ensure success with our purpose. God has a reason for putting us in these trying times. We have a purpose during the difficult events as well as the joyful ones. These purposes give meaning to the human experience. They provide order to the chaos that surrounds us and gives us a sense of accomplishment each day.

The reasons I write a chapter for military wives are twofold: one, to honor the sacrifice and strength of the military spouse. Military spouses are awe-inspiring. God gives them incredible strength to get through hardships and do it with a smile and grace. I am humbled to be a part of a community of military spouses that share a belief that they are a part of something much bigger than themselves. Each time a spouse marries into the military, they give us something of themselves and have to realize that career, time, and identity has now become a part of what their soldier is doing. It is often done selflessly.

Second, I write about military spouses because there is a lesson for us all going through trying times. We all have the ability to take conflict, adversity, and tragedy and turn it into something more than ourselves. Military spouses are not the only spouses that are separated from their loved ones for something greater than themselves. We all have moments when we need to learn to keep our families together when we are faced with challenges from work and the world. This is God's purpose for us. We are not here for ourselves. Even the dying man has a gift to be given to the world at large; it may be your call to figure out what that message will be. *Our adversities provide an opportunity in which we can set new goals in order to become stronger individuals and stronger believers.* As we develop into stronger believers, we are able to lift up those around us and create a stronger community of God. We can do this through physical exercise, prayer, meditation, and healthful choices in our individual lives, for our families and for our communities.

The military spouse is never alone in his/her purpose. You are not either.

THOUGHTS TO PONDER:

1. How do you perceive adversity, trying times, or separations from your family?

2. Can you think of a healthy approach to your adversity that would make you a stronger person, individual, family, or community?

3. What goal would you like to set through your times of adversity that will give you a sense of accomplishment, peace, and purpose?

See, I have set before you today life and prosperity, death and adversity.
—Deuteronomy 30:15

DAY 29   Steps taken: _____   Miles journeyed: _____

Exercise chosen: _____

Spiritual thoughts: _____

_____

_____

_____

Feelings: _____

_____

_____

_____

DAY 30 Christ Walk Dads

BIBLICAL BIG IDEA #30

Listen, children, to a father's instruction, and be attentive, that you may gain insight. —Proverbs 4:1

I wrote a day dedicated to moms. I feel equally called to write a day for dads. It may be the time that my life is in, but parenthood weighs heavily on my mind and heart! I want to jump right in and say that I want this chapter to be inclusive. I want to address this for parents who are parenting individually or as a couple. If I make a *faux pas* along the way, I ask your forgiveness in advance. My experience with parenting is as a married couple. Is this the only way to parent? Certainly not. I might have gotten a taste of single parenting after my husband's last deployment, but it doesn't give me the right to call myself a single parent. However, I want to do my best to recognize that parenting, fatherhood, grandparenthood, etc., comes in all sorts of shapes and sizes.

While parenting may be done individually as a "single parent" or as a couple in a traditional marriage or other arrangement, at the end of the day, it takes a male and female to make a child. There are roles for both men and women in the parenting of children. This does not mean that one is more important than the other. This just means there are different roles. Some people have both a mom and a dad; other people get their experience with a "father figure" or "mother figure" from different people. So when I refer to "father" in the text below, I am trying to describe the role model that shapes a child outside of just mom.

Being a mom or dad means to be fully engaged and committed to sharing Christ's love with our kids. This goes beyond the biological. We made this promise when we brought our children to be baptized and affirmed the Baptismal Covenant in the Book of Common Prayer. Whether we are single parenting or co-parenting, or a role model at church, in school, or in the community, we all have the opportunity to parent children. We shape our sons and daughters through the love we give them, which shapes them to be leaders in God's land and their place in the world.

Fathers, grandfathers, and father figures are so very important to children. Fathers are role models for healthy habits in body, mind, and spirit. Most children see their fathers as heroes, as omnipotent beings who can do no wrong and must know everything. Because our children see their fathers in this light, a father is in a unique position to show his children how to exercise, eat healthy, pray, share their feelings, and learn continuously. When children see that both men and women have healthy habits, then habits transcend gender. All of these modelled behaviors are tools we want to teach our kids to help them become productive members of society. Parents who are not afraid to show their children these things, speak frankly, and *listen* are providing their children with a safe environment in which to practice healthy living mind, body, and soul.

Parents can take a page from God's book by proclaiming to their children, "This is my child with whom I am well pleased!" Children need to hear they are special; that their parent(s) are proud of them; and that there is an important place in the world for them to do God's work. Parents need to work together on teaching boundaries, and rules, and what is right and wrong. We must work together to teach to love one another. We can first do this by loving each other and showing loving relationships to our children.

Dads, and now increasingly more moms, have the burden of leaving their kids to support the family. I took for granted that my husband could leave the house and go to work but did not consider how hard it was for him to leave the kids and miss them. This was especially apparent when he had to leave them for long periods of time. While it is easy for me to moan and groan that he is gone and not having to deal with the whining, crying, and screaming, I tend to forget that he misses them greatly each day. I certainly do not feel equipped to do the parenting role on my own and I am eternally thankful that I do not have to do this alone as others may have to do.

I am an optimist. I really believe that both moms and dads are just trying to do what is best for their families. Is this always the case? No, but I think that there are more people who are trying their best than there are not. Part of doing one's best is providing for a family. Part of providing for that family is going to work. However, it is important that we are mindful of a work-life-family-spiritual balance. Just as for moms, it is important that dads take the time to prioritize prayer, family time, exercise time, and healthful habits, even as they go to work. Parents are partners in this endeavor to raise children and we have to take the time to talk about how to move forward, what to do to create this family, and how to address the problems and tribulations that arise. When parents do not talk, discuss, or listen, problems begin to occur. Both parties feel neglected and bitter and problems grow exponentially when they are not addressed in a safe environment.

My husband and I have used various methods over the last few years to ensure we continue to talk through trying to raise kids, manage the house, have careers, and raise a Christian family. We have used the "floor method" from PREP (Planned Relationship Enhancement Program) as well as attending the Worldwide Marriage Encounter (http://wwme. org/). We found the guidance from Dr. Gary Chapman's *The Five Love Languages: The Secret to Love That Lasts* to be extremely helpful. What we both learned is that whatever method you want to use, the bottom line is that you need to communicate regularly with your partner and express the concerns that you may otherwise be afraid to voice, in a safe environment. If spouses are not taking the time to communicate, then communication breaks down. When you don't communicate, you don't generate the relationship and love between two people that is so important in showing God's love to kids! And if you are anything like me, when you don't communicate, you have conversations in your head against your spouse, taking one small issue and blowing it up to many issues. Somehow the laundry on the floor evolves into every reason the spouse does not care enough, love you enough, or understand you enough. Yet, if I have not taken the time to discuss the laundry on the floor, I have not given my spouse the opportunity to change or respond to my frustration.

Spouses also need to remind each other regularly why they fell in love. Most people fell in love at some point in their relationship. Most people get married because they fell in love. Where there is love there is God, and that is something valuable and precious to treasure and nurture over time. Unfortunately, over time, love may feel like it got old. I do not believe that the love got old, but we do get very familiar with that love and it does not seem as new or shiny as when we first met our spouses. Through communication and devoting time to one another, you can find ways to feed that fire. I have come to realize that when I am supporting my husband and we are working on the love we have, he becomes a better father. I know that I need reassurance that I am a good mom. It is normal that fathers also need that reassurance that they are doing a good job as well.

Not every family can have both a mother and a father. A parent may be challenged to provide these examples on his or her own. God can be the father to the child if there is a missing father, as well as a mother if there is a missing mother. It is up to that parent, though, to bring the child to God and allow opportunities for God to help raise that child. And let's face it, no matter how "perfect" a job we may (or may not) do as a parent, children will find fault with the way a parent parents. Children will take things they thought you did right and mimic them. Other actions, they will swear they will do differently when they have their own children. No child will think his or her parents did the perfect parenting job. One day, our kids will learn how difficult the parenting job can be!

As a mother or a father, we must know that we are not alone in this endeavor. If we raise our kids with love, then we are doing the best job we can. If we raise our kids with love, then we are putting God (and God's commandment) first in our parenting. If we place God first, then every parent will have a role model in which to equip their children with a life-long loving family.

THOUGHTS TO PONDER

1. Do you feel comfortable as a parent, as a role model for your children?

2. Are there opportunities for you to model better behavior for your children?

3. Are you and your spouse communicating so you are raising children together?

Everyone who believes that Jesus is the Christ has been born of God, and everyone who loves the parent loves the child. By this we know that we love the children of God, when we love God and obey his commandments. For the love of God is this, that we obey his commandments. —1 John 5:1–3

DAY 30 Steps taken: _____ Miles journeyed: _____

Exercise chosen: _____

Spiritual thoughts: _____

_____

_____

Feelings: _____

_____

_____

_____

When Jesus Carries You

BIBLICAL BIG IDEA #31

And the power of the Lord was with [Jesus] to heal. Just then some men came, carrying a paralyzed man on a bed. They were trying to bring him in and lay him before Jesus; but finding no way to bring him in because of the crowd, they went up on the roof and let him down with his bed through the tiles into the middle of the crowd in front of Jesus. —Luke 5:17b–19

I will be honest. I find that I have a body that frustrates me at every turn. I have nagging chronic illness, injuries, and diseases. I do not have anything that is tragic and life-threatening, but my body challenges me daily on what I think it should do versus what it can do. It can be exhausting, mentally and physically, to deal with chronic illnesses, especially when so many aspects of the disease seem out of my control. The good news is that mounds of evidence and scientific study say prayer, physical exercise, and good nutrition can support chronic and acute disease management.

Simply put, when you take care of your body well, the illness will have less impact on your activities of daily living and pursuit of physical fitness goals. Does this mean there will not be stumbling blocks along the way? No. On the contrary, anyone who has an illness knows that you have your good days and bad. On the bad days, you do what you can. On the good days you go for the gold and be all you can be. Through both types of days you pray for strength and support. On the good days we give thanks to God that we were able to meet our goals. No matter which type of day, I believe that the grace of God carries us through these times. Just as the poem "Footprints" attests, there are days that Jesus carries us through our Christ Walk, when we ourselves cannot.

When I was losing my hearing as a child, there was a woman in our church who told my mom that she needed to take me to a faith healer so that I would be cured. This did not sit well with my mom, and over the years I have often pondered that perhaps my faith in God's ability to heal is not as strong as I think it is in my heart. I am often quick to think, "We'll take care of the worldly ills, God, as long as you are taking care of heavenly needs." The Bible is filled with stories of Jesus' healing, with strong messages that if you have faith, you will be healed.

And to the centurion Jesus said, "Go; let it be done for you according to your faith." And the servant was healed in that hour. —Matthew 8:13

and

When Jesus heard this, he replied, "Do not fear. Only believe, and she will be saved." —Luke 8:50

and

Now many signs and wonders were done among the people through the apostles.—Acts 5:12a

I feared that because I was not healed and my body was not whole, my faith was not good enough. Perhaps I needed to have more faith to have the miracle of a whole and healthy body. Fear can sow doubt in the soul. My fear has led me to question God's mercy and grace. Fear is a conduit to sin.

I read the stories in the Bible on healing, and the doubt that creeps into my psyche causes me to think that maybe I really do not believe that God will heal me. This is a very uncomfortable thought. If I define healing as solely the restoration of my hearing as I heard as a child, then I have put limits on God's definition of healing. Instead, six months following my deafness, cochlear implants became approved for children less than six months of age. I had no hearing. We prayed for hearing and cochlear implants became available. God works in mysterious ways. It may not be how I first imaged healing, but it was still healing. And now I do hear!

This was my miracle. I believe in miracles and have seen many happen. Miracles are often not what you think they will be. Miracles are works of God, not people. Therefore a miracle may not be perceived in human terms as a miracle. I have lived long enough to realize that God's view of the world differs from my own. God's perception of healing and growth are not necessarily what we anticipate. I do not get angry at God about the loss of my hearing, or about why I have autoimmune diseases. I share my anger with God because I know that God is the only one who can take my anger and remove it from me so that I can move on. From there, I am able to continue God's work in the world. Is this not healing? Yes, there are times that I wistfully wish that I did not wear hearing aids. They can be cumbersome. I am dependent on batteries. I am deaf at night, and I am deaf in the water. I often wish that sometimes it wasn't so easy to miss conversations with my children, and yet, my hearing loss made me into the person I am today. I do not feel less whole because I hear less. On the contrary, God has made me all the stronger from my loss. This is a type of healing and growth that I would not have had if God had pushed a magic button and I had hearing again.

Sometimes the self doubt comes back and I wonder, "Am I simply trying to rationalize why I was not wholly healed from my prayers to include a full set of working ears? Is that not what the Bible is saying to me to have faith and God will heal you? What exactly is God trying to say here?" What exactly is healing?

Recently, I found a lump in one breast, which was confirmed by my doctor. This started a round of mammograms and ultrasounds I was not yet fully prepared to undergo at my age. A friend and a cousin were diagnosed with breast cancer in their twenties and thirties, respectively, and I began to worry that I was going to be one of those statistics. I made it through the mammogram fine, but as I lay half-dressed by myself on the ultrasound table, I could not keep the fears at bay. A self-proclaimed worrier, no matter how much I pray and practice, a litany of what-ifs parade through my mind when I am presented with the unknown. When in the dark, vulnerable and alone, fear makes every worry larger.

As I lay on the table and prayed that I did not have cancer, I was again struck by the stories that if you have enough faith in God to heal you, then you will be healed. In that moment I was very angry; I felt like these passages in the Bible were challenging my faith when I was most vulnerable. I believe in God's mercy, wisdom, omniscience, and omnipotence. I believe that God is my strong rock and a castle to keep me safe. If I am not healed and have cancer (or any of my other illnesses), would I then stop believing in God? A faith that is contingent upon healing or removing disease seems like a rather weak faith. But my faith is stronger because I know that *even if a disease of the world* continues in my body; my soul will forever be healed by God's grace. There is a place for me "with all the company of heaven," because I have been healed by God's grace—even with a rotten body.

If I continue to believe that my faith solely relies on the mercy of God to heal that disease, then he also must make minute-by-minute judgments on children getting killed, wars, famine, earthquakes, or other disasters. I do not believe this. I do not believe that God picks and chooses where to intervene in the world. I believe we are called to have a relationship with God despite the ills in the world. The world is what we have made it as humans. God gave us freedom of choice. God gives us the opportunity to make the choice to live as Christians, to love one another, no matter what is going on around us. Even in the midst of tragedy, we have the opportunity to make the decision to love.

God's grace will get us through these times on our flawed earth. The love we share with one another represents God's grace on earth and makes those flawed times precious. The way we approach this time is how we build our temple mind, body, and spirit. This is our opportunity to prepare ourselves for the time in which we are with God in heaven, and illness is not something we will ever have to worry over again.

You may be ill. Like me, you may suffer from a physical chronic illness. Perhaps you have been stricken with an acute disease, cancer, or heart disease, and that is requiring you to look at your life completely differently. Perhaps you are like my father who is afflicted by mental illness. With a relationship with God, you can find healing in your soul and spirit through faith. With faith in God, it does not matter what is going on with your worldly body—it will do what you need it to do for the time you have it—but your spiritual body will be stronger than ever before.

And that is my belief on the healing that God provides with faith. It is healing, just not what you think it may be.

THOUGHTS TO PONDER

1. Do you feel that you are stuck physically, mentally, or spiritually, because God won't heal you?

2. Where do you find God's healing? Is it what you expected?

3. Even though your body, mind, and spirit might not be where you want them to be, what strengths has God given you to make change?

Happy are those who consider the poor; the LORD *delivers them in the day of trouble.* —Psalm 41:1

DAY 31   Steps taken: _____   Miles journeyed: _____

Exercise chosen: _____

Spiritual thoughts: _____

_____

_____

_____

_____

Feelings: _____

_____

_____

_____

_____

Living Simply

BIBLICAL BIG IDEA #32

A tranquil mind gives life to the flesh, but passion makes the bones rot. —Proverbs 14:30

For anyone who knows me, the irony of the focus of this day's reflection is not lost. I am TERRIBLE at living simply. I pack entirely too much in my day, I bite off more than I can chew, and I look to myself to be a superwoman in the world rather than letting God be the superhero. I can be very preoccupied with the world's concept of what I *should* be doing as a wife and mother. I should manage a career, I should raise two angels, I should take care of the house and the kids, I should be active in church, I should work out every day, I should avoid processed foods, I should give more, do more, act more, dress more, look more and more, more, more, more. . . .

I am tired just reading that sentence! I am baffled that with more and more conveniences the world seems all the more complex and demanding. We clean more than ever even though we have vacuum cleaners, washing machines, and dish washers. These contraptions were designed so that we would have more time to spend with our families and enjoy the world God gave us, and yet we do not. Everyone works harder and harder these days, and I constantly wonder, "Is the world a better place?"

Overall, as an optimist, I truly believe the world is a better place. However, with the demands of the world and the constant pursuit of more, more, more, we tend to forget to separate out the demands of the world and focus on what God calls us to do.

On Day 5 we completed an exercise in which we described the three most important things in our lives. I have told you that mine are God, family, and health. When I am not living simply by adding, more, more, and more into my life, I have let these priorities stray from my life. More, more, and more adds more stress into my life, which is neither good for my health nor my family. Adding more and more tends to push God to the end of my priority list instead of keeping him at the front.

What I have to remind myself when I am not living simply and the more, more, more is getting the better of me, is to refocus on my priority list and what is MOST important in my life. This brings me back into focus and I find it much easier to separate the activities that are chaff from the activities that are wheat in my life. When I am focusing on those goals, it becomes easier to begin to discard convenience foods, unwholesome choices, a rat race of a career, and other things that are not a part of my simple life. I am healthy because I focus on building my body to be stronger for my priorities. It is an empty trophy if I focus on my vanity, if I have not done it in pursuit of something greater than me.

There is so much we worry about and take on that is really unnecessary to live a Christlike life. Recently, I contemplated a Facebook update along the lines of, "Dear God, please do not be afraid to use a 2x4 on my head. It's very thick and I seem to need a reminder of the important things in life far too often." Living simply means to focus on your priorities. Put God first and include your health as a part of your godly practice. You will begin needing less in your life as you make God part of your everyday practice, not just on Sunday. Christ Walk is every day.

Living simply will also lead to healthier choices in life. Focusing on the foods from the earth instead of from the process mill will ensure the richest nutrients enter your body. Taking a bike ride or a walk instead of a drive ensures activity for your body. It takes care of the earth with less exhaust released into the atmosphere and reduces the amount you spend on gas for your car. Reducing waste and packaged products ensures you have less clutter in your life. When you purchase less packaged and processed food, you reduce waste in your house as well as spending less money on food that is bad for you. Buying only what you need teaches your children not to waste money and to save for the most important things. Choosing to walk, run, bike, eat, and worship locally is good for you, good for the earth, good for the community, and builds a sense of wellbeing that you will never regret.

The more you learn to live simply, the less you seem to need in your life. The less you have to fill up the spaces in your life with "more, more, and more," the more room you have for God to enter those spaces to share your Christ Walk wherever you may go.

May the God of hope fill you with all joy and peace in believing, so that you may abound in hope by the power of the Holy Spirit. —Romans 15:13

If you have filled your life with the "more, more, more," then there will be no places for the Holy Spirit to fill you to overflowing. When the

Holy Spirit is allowed to overflow in you, it flows to those around you, thereby passing God's grace to others.

THOUGHTS TO PONDER

1. How can you live more simply?

2. What are you filling your life with "more, more, more" that could be replaced with time for God?

3. If you were overflowing with the Holy Spirit and filled with God's love, where would it overflow in your life to others?

For this reason I bow my knees before the Father, from whom every family in heaven and on earth takes its name. I pray that, according to the riches of his glory, he may grant that you may be strengthened in your inner being with power through his Spirit, and that Christ may dwell in your hearts through faith, as you are being rooted and grounded in love. I pray that you may have the power to comprehend, with all the saints, what is the breadth and length and height and depth, and to know the love of Christ that surpasses knowledge, so that you may be filled with all the fullness of God. —Ephesians 3:14–19

DAY 32   Steps taken: _____   Miles journeyed: _____

Exercise chosen: _____

Spiritual thoughts: _____

_____

_____

_____

Feelings: _____

_____

_____

_____

DAY 33 Reevaluating Goals

BIBLICAL BIG IDEA #33

Our hope is that, as your faith increases, our sphere of action among you may be greatly enlarged, so that we may proclaim the good news in lands beyond you.
—2 Corinthians 10:15b–16a

So we are nearing the end of our forty-day journey. Perhaps you are coming close to the end of your goal. Perhaps you are feeling guilty because you have not walked as far as you thought you would. Perhaps events occurred during the forty days that were beyond your control and have you wondering, "Where do I go from here?"

Journeys and goals do not end once you reach your initial goal. Journeys and goals are times where we learn to grow into our capabilities. Perhaps you took on too much too soon. Does this mean you stop and do not continue your journey? No, you will continue this journey until you are strong and able, doing God's work as your body calls you to do. If you are excelling with your initial goal and it does not seem to be challenging you, then maybe it is time for you to reevaluate and challenge yourself to something new. Just because we walked a mile today does not mean we cannot try to walk two miles tomorrow. Similarly, just because we gave $10.00 to the church yesterday does not mean we do not look for ways to give more in the future.

Goals are not the end. God's expectation of us as Christians does not end with one goal or deed. Being a Christian is a lifelong expectation of giving and sacrifice. When we give our bodies over to do the work of God, the benefits and joy we reap is beyond understanding. Likewise, the health of the body is a lifelong pursuit. Although we may have reached our goal to run three miles, lose ten pounds, or reduce our blood pressure by ten points, it does not mean that the life of the couch potato gets to return. It was a very shocking realization to me that in order to pursue a certain level of health or lose a certain number of pounds, I ultimately was going to have to do this for the rest of my life. The weight, fatigue, and lack of endurance or strength will creep back on to our bodies if we sit back and do not continue to exercise. We tend to focus on ourselves and our faults rather than the great things we can do with these bodies that God gave us when we are sick and unfit.

Similarly, once we take on the Christian mantle, we are not called to sit back on our laurels. On the contrary, the Bible states very clearly to be wary of resting too comfortably on our achievements, as this is an opportunity for sin to creep into our lives.

At that time, I will search Jerusalem with lamps, and I will punish the people who rest complacently on their dregs, those who say in their hearts, "The Lord will not do good, nor will he do harm." —Zephaniah 1:12

God will do amazing things through you if you give God the chance to do that work with you. While we are only saved by God's grace, the Cross comes with expectations of behavior, duty, and love that transcend a lifetime. We do not go on vacation from being Christian, nor do we take vacations from our health. The consequences could be quite severe.

Having said that, everyone has goals, and everyone has goals that they do not meet. A goal may be to get out of bed for the day, and that is truly an excellent goal if this is a struggle! Goals will continue to change each day and each moment as we are faced with the challenges of the world around us. Perhaps you have had amazing success with your initial goal. Perhaps you have journeyed the miles to Jerusalem and back. The good news is that there are many other journeys in the Bible to tackle. Perhaps your next goal could be to run or walk the miles to Rome over the course of the year and study Paul's journeys to spread Christianity amongst the early church.

Your spiritual goals can support your physical goals. We should challenge ourselves to go further, to work harder, and to be all that we can be. In the Army, they call this Army Strong. In the church, we should be God Strong. We become God Strong through God's grace to live a healthy life mind, body, and spirit.

With great power the apostles gave their testimony to the resurrection of the Lord Jesus, and great grace was upon them all. —Acts 4:33

God's grace in us will make us God Strong.

If you were unable to meet your goal, it is a great idea to reevaluate. Perhaps you bit off more than you could chew. Or perhaps you need to prayerfully consider what God is calling you to do with your body and discuss with a spiritual or fitness advisor how to get there. Taking a leap towards a healthy life when you have never been healthy is often daunting. And it is difficult to remind yourself that doing the best you can do for the day, may be the best you can do it, *and it is okay*. Remember this is not the pursuit of a Hollywood body. This is the pursuit of a healthy temple for God.

To be renewed in the spirit of your minds, and to clothe yourselves with the new self, created according to the likeness of God in true righteousness and holiness. So then, putting away falsehood, let us all speak the truth to our neighbors, for we are all members of one another. —Ephesians 4:23–25

This body you have is God's body. This individual body is a part of a greater body of God's people. The body of God in the world is the church. It is a righteous body and a holy body and you are called to take care of it. It is our responsibility for taking care of our physical body as well as the body of the church. We need to put off our excuses and justifications for our poor choices. Every day we need to pray about making the right choices for a healthier body. I believe that any time you repent the sins of the body, God will redeem that body. God is ever faithful, ever merciful, and ever patient. Each day that we might not meet our Christ Walk goal is okay, because, through God's forgiving nature, we have the next day to set a new goal and challenge to do that much more.

Through God's grace I am given God's peace, which passes any understanding I may have. I am awed and comforted that no matter how hard I try, it is only through God's grace that I am able to go farther, try harder, do more, or make a difference. It is only through God's grace that I am even attempting this book! Through a leap of faith, I stepped out of my comfort zone to try something new and take on a new challenge. Even if you are in a wheelchair, or a walker, or have other challenges of the body, you too can take a leap of faith and God's grace will take you through. I have faith that there is more in store for your body than you ever thought possible. God's work is not done with our bodies until we have passed on into God's care at death.

Sailors have a saying about themselves: "Sailors don't have plans, they have intentions." That is because when sailing, you are at the mercy of the winds and sea, so sailors try to focus more on the journey and less on the goal. As with sailing, if circumstances outside your control change your goal, you can still make the journey worthwhile.

Do not fear. Do not become complacent. There is more to this journey than the goal you first set. Try a new journey. Take a leap of faith. Set a new goal or attempt an old goal again. Because God has redeemed us, we have many chances to get it right!

THOUGHTS TO PONDER

1. Are you on track to complete your Christ Walk goal? What will be your new goal if you cannot complete your original goal?

2. Are you disappointed that you will not meet your goal? Have you considered keeping at it after the end of your forty-day challenge?

3. Either way, what is your next Christ Walk goal? What do you need to do differently this next time around to be successful?

Not that I have already obtained this or have already reached the goal; but I press on to make it my own, because Christ Jesus has made me his own.
—Philippians 3:12

DAY 33 Steps taken: _____ Miles journeyed: _____

Exercise chosen: _____

Spiritual thoughts: _____

_____

_____

_____

Feelings: _____

_____

_____

_____

34 Making Mind, Body, and Spiritual Health Your Priority

BIBLICAL BIG IDEA #34

Always carrying in the body the death of Jesus, so that the life of Jesus may also be made visible in our bodies.
—2 Corinthians 4:10

Early on in this challenge, on Day 5, we discussed the most important things in your life. You would think that the most important things in your life would easily become those things that are a priority in life. I *know* that your physical, mental, and spiritual health are important to you. You have picked up this book and challenged yourself to change your body and your spirit and to walk with God for forty days. You have marched on through thick and thin during this challenge to put one foot in front of the other and to make yourself "God Strong" during this time. But I imagine it has been a struggle. Even when we know that physical and spiritual health are so important to us, it is easy to let the world take over, and these things that are important to us get pushed to the end of the list instead of the beginning. I know this. I am a victim of this paradox myself. Heck, if I had had all my priorities in order, this book may have been written much faster than it was. And yet, things that matter little creep their way into my world and my work-life-spirit balance becomes off-center. I become grumpy and irritable, and I wonder what is wrong. When I take a moment to reflect and consider, I always discover that I have let my priorities get out of order.

We must remind ourselves of our priorities continually:

You therefore, beloved, since you are forewarned, beware that you are not be carried away with the error of the lawless and lose your own stability.
—2 Peter 3:17

The world will forever be knocking over our priorities and trying to set them askew. There are many tools at your disposal to keep your priorities and goals at the forefront of your mind:

1. Pray.
Pray without ceasing. —1 Thessalonians 5:17

2. Develop a plan with God.
The human mind plans the way, but the LORD directs the steps.
—Proverbs 16:9

3. Make a list of what you want to do.
"If you do well, will you not be accepted? And if you do not do well, sin is lurking at the door; its desire is for you, but you must master it."
—Genesis 4:7

4. Schedule your priorities *first.*
They gave themselves first to the Lord and, by the will of God, to us.
—2 Corinthians 8:5b

5. Ask for forgiveness when you mess up.
Remember then from what you have fallen; repent, and do the works you did at first. If not, I will come to you and remove your lampstand from its place, unless you repent. —Revelation 2:5

6. Because God is merciful, forgive yourself as God forgives you.
The LORD will fulfill his purpose for me; your steadfast love, O LORD, endures forever. Do not forsake the work of your hands. —Psalm 138:8

7. Because the Lord does not abandon the works of his hands, get up and try again.
I know your works—your love, faith, service, and patient endurance. I know that your last works are greater than the first. —Revelation 2:19

You have come this far; you will continue to walk with God and continue to make God's work and your health a priority in your life. One spark of change creates a lifetime of ripples that will continue to move priorities in the right place in your life. The more you practice these priorities, the more they become a part of you and your life, and soon Christ Walk will be a part of every step you take in your life!

THOUGHTS TO PONDER

1. What is my priority list?

2. Am I sticking with it?

3. What do I need to revaluate?

4. Where do I need to schedule my priorities better so that mind, body, and spiritual health come first?

The best of the first fruits of your ground you shall bring to the house of the LORD *your God.* —Exodus 34:26

DAY 34   Steps taken: _____   Miles journeyed: _____

Exercise chosen: _____

Spiritual thoughts: _____

_____

_____

_____

Feelings: _____

_____

_____

_____

Being Inspired

BIBLICAL BIG IDEA #35

But I do not count my life of any value to myself, if only I may finish my course and the ministry I received from the Lord Jesus, to testify to the good news of God's grace. —Acts 20:24

What brings inspiration to you? I am constantly inspired. I believe I am inspired by the work of the Spirit within me and in those around me. Because I believe that there is a God-spark in all of us, I believe that everyone has the capability of being inspired and being inspirational. Those that inspire me physically are those who have run the race no matter their challenges. Individuals who pick themselves up after tragedy are inspirational. Many people do not believe that these acts are miracles from God. I believe it is the work of the Spirit of God in the world around us that plants these seeds of inspiration. Although we may be presented with challenges of the *world*, we will always be tethered to the inspiration of the divine through the God-spark in all of us. When we choose to love one another as God loved us, we are the very vehicles of God's grace and inspiration of the world. What is more inspiring than loving one another?

There is a young mother who lost her soldier-husband shortly after their third child was born. Her inspiration was to run; not run away, but to run in honor and memory of the love that they shared. Her physical endurance and strength brought other women who had also lost their soldiers to run as well. "Wear Blue: Run to Remember" advocates, "We are a living memory to the soldier, to the fallen and to their families." This organization started because of the love two people built. This is inspiring. Where there is love, there is God, even in loss. Learn more at: http://www.wearblueruntoremember.org.

Love gives strength as well as inspiration. I believe that one reason my father did not die from his debilitating stroke was because of the love he had for my mother. He was not ready to let her go. I believe that my mother survived her bone marrow transplant because of the love of friends, family and God that lifted her up and the prayers that wrapped her in comfort. The presence of God in those who are dying is inspiring to me. We do not know what happens in the last seconds of one's life, but I believe that God is there.

I called to the LORD out of my distress, and he answered me; out of the belly of Sheol I cried, and you heard my voice. —Jonah 2:2

I believe that when we call on God, God is there. I am inspired that God is there for me.

As we begin to wrap up our forty-day journey towards healthy living, I am calling on you to be inspired to continue this journey. Your goals of walking, running, biking, swimming, *actively living*, should not end here. Your task now is to be inspired to continue on. God always gives us opportunities to try again, even if we fail the first, second, or third time. Redemption is about renewal; we can continue to try for greater goals of healthy living through the power of the Spirit.

You may choose to repeat this book. There are a number of walking/running mileage goals contained in the appendices to take you to the next level. There are goals for beginner, intermediate, or advanced levels, and there are many routes for each level to inspire you in a new direction. Perhaps you will build your spiritual study around one of the new routes to understand the journey that Jesus and the disciples were taking as they traversed what we call the Holy Land today. Perhaps you have transformed yourself to take on a new challenge to run for a spiritual goal, perhaps to raise money for one of your church's mission funds. I have never been more inspired than when my goals are built around strengthening myself while doing something for others. I am never more lifted up than when my time, talent, and treasure are spent in building others up and I feel stronger, healthier, and more alive with this inspiration coursing through me.

You were inspired to take on this forty-day challenge, but it is important that the challenge does not stop here. God forgives us when we turn away from our unhealthy choices, and our acts of repentance bring us closer to the right choices. God will continually inspire us over the course of a lifetime to do the right things for our bodies and to use them for the greater good. When the flow of inspiration seems to be running low or missing, we should turn to prayer, study, and meditation to allow ourselves to be open. God will answer the question, "Where do I go from here?" The answer may be something you did not expect and in a time when you were not ready.

*Then he came to the disciples and found them sleeping; and he said to Peter,
"So, could you not stay awake with me one hour? Stay awake and pray that
you may not come into the time of trial; the spirit indeed is willing, but the flesh
is weak."* —Matthew 26:40–41

If we are actively engaged in our spirituality and health, the inspiration
will flow more easily. Our repetitive behaviors will condition our bodies
to be open to that inspiration that will take us to the next level of health,
wellness, and spirituality.

One of my "a-ha" moments with my health came when I realized
that the changes I made in my diet, exercise, prayer, and health were not
short-term changes. Just because I lost the weight or fended off the disease did not mean that I got to go back to my bad habits. Rather, the light
bulb went off that this was a *lifelong* commitment to my physical health,
to my spiritual health, to my family's health, and to my relationship with
God. These changes were not a quick fix. These changes needed to be
with me forever. While God will *always* be there, I realized that to feel
that relationship, it was *I* who was going to have to continue to work
on my behaviors and engage myself in that relationship. God does not
demand from us a relationship, but it is a far more fulfilling life when that
relationship is fully active and mutual. I am inspired and fulfilled with this
lifelong pursuit of a healthy life. Each day that I take on this challenge to
a healthier life, body, mind, and soul, I am reminded that there is something that I can always work on to do better.

We do not retire from our health or our relationship with God. God
will always be there to inspire us at any point in our life to go to the next
level. If a sixty-five- or seventy-five-year-old can train for a marathon, we,
too, have limitless possibilities no matter our stage in life. This is God's
grace at work through us. Aren't you inspired?

THOUGHTS TO PONDER

1. What do you find inspiring?

2. Where will you seek inspiration?

3. What are some possible ways that God might be calling you to be
inspired in your life?

*All scripture is inspired by God and is useful for teaching, for reproof, for
correction, and for training in righteousness, so that everyone who belongs to
God may be proficient, equipped for every good work.* —2 Timothy 3:16–17

DAY 35 Steps taken: _____   Miles journeyed: _____

Exercise chosen: _____

Spiritual thoughts: _____

_____

_____

_____

_____

Feelings: _____

_____

_____

_____

_____

Going to the Next Level

BIBLICAL BIG IDEA #36

*My brothers and sisters, whenever you face trials of any kind,
consider it nothing but joy, because you know that the testing
of your faith produces endurance.* —James 1:2–3

So now that we are inspired, and we know that the journey does not end at day forty, we need to take it to the next level. There will always be some sort of work for us to do in the world, no matter our health or capabilities. *Everyone* has a contribution to make to the world that we live in because we are all members of the Body of Christ. The work you may be called to do as a marathoner may be different from the work called of the individual trying to walk a mile for the first time. Both individuals have something they are called to do.

When I am stumped about where I go from here, I often have to sit back and take stock. I need to congratulate myself on how far I have come. Even though there is still more road to follow and improvements to be made, just trying to meet my goals each day is an accomplishment in itself. If I look back on myself during the past ten years, I am more cardiovascular fit than in my college years, although I do weigh a few pounds more. I have challenged my body in ways I never thought possible, even though I now have more grey hairs and wrinkles. I wish I had started living a life of health and fitness at an earlier age because it is so much easier to get fit when you're younger. This is why I encourage parents to build a life of health and fitness in their children while they are young. While you *can* learn to play soccer (or any other sport) at any age in your life, it is a lot easier to train your body to respond to new physical demands when those muscles are still young and developing.

My parents were not huge athletes growing up. My mom did not play sports, and while my dad played a number of sports, fitness was not something they learned as being a lifelong endeavor. My dad did not think that he needed to keep up with his physical fitness upon retirement from the Navy, and like many sailors and soldiers before him, all of a sudden the weight began creeping on. Coming from the South, my mom was raised that "women do not sweat, they perspire." This of course does not lend to making vigorous exercise and physical fitness a priority. My parents were raised by a generation for whom physical activity was a part of their everyday lives. They did not have to "work out" to stay fit. Being active and fit was just what they did *to* work and live. On top of that, my parents are cerebral people. They tend to gravitate to the arts, music, and literature. What a fantastic education this provided to my brother and me! However, this left me to teach myself how to add physical fitness into my life. Thank God my mom made home-cooked meals for us with fresh ingredients! Otherwise I would have had a double whammy against me as I learned to build a healthy body.

Learning physical exercise in our youth is really important. Just like losing weight or changing bad health habits, we have to retrain our muscles and bodies when taking on new tasks. During the adolescent years, those muscles are primed to be developed into new capabilities. Let your children explore a variety of different activities—do not force them to become Little League all-stars if their joy is in kung fu. The early years are great for exploring a wide variety of physical opportunities. As children grow older, they will find something on which to focus their talents and that may be walking quietly on their own. That is okay. Not all individuals are social athletes. Some of our children will be into solitary endeavors. The trick is to give them options. We should provide opportunities each day for them to be physically active.

Strategy one is to explore a variety of physical activities with your children. Continue to wear your pedometer as you all try out something new and continue to track the number of miles and steps you take each day. If you do not have children, try something new that you never considered before. Stories of sixty- and seventy-year-olds running races for the first time humble me. I will never forget getting passed during my first half marathon by a seventy-five-year-old gentleman who had a shirt on that said, "Can you keep up with me at my age? Seventy-five years and counting." Or eighty-year-olds jumping out of planes! And people who are in wheelchairs or use walkers getting out and moving anyway!

There are additional benefits to this trying something new. When we have been exercising in a certain way for a certain period of time, our muscles get used to the work we are doing. If we are trying to lose weight or improve our fitness, we can plateau with repetition of the same type of exercise over and over. It is important to mix things up so that our bodies do not get bored and the muscles are always learning new ways to move and work. Remember that every fifteen minutes of whatever activity you choose is worth one Christ Walk mile. This way you can continue your Christ Walk experience and still mix it up!

Strategy two is similar. You have now been walking with a pedometer (or biking, running, swimming, or doing aerobics) for close to forty days. Look back over the progress that you have made these past few weeks. Grab a calculator and take an average of steps you have completed to this point: Add all your steps (or miles) together; divide by 36 (today is Day 36). Or add up your total number of steps or miles and divide by the number of days you have completed. This will be your average daily distance for the program. Your next strategy would be to set a goal to add 2,000 steps to this average for next forty-day period. If you are averaging 15 to 20 miles of activity over the last forty days, see if you can increase that mileage to a safe level by adding no more than 10% per week. It is important to realize here that everyone has different capabilities and goals. Someone who is an athlete may be able to safely ramp up his or her miles at a rate higher than an individual taking on exercise for the first time.

If you are unsure how to increase your level of fitness, find a fitness professional to give you guidance tailored to your specific fitness level. Likewise, even if you are a physical fitness stud, a fitness professional can teach you new tricks for taking your fitness to the next level. It is important to first realize that everyone is different and everyone needs to tailor their changes to their fitness level. These are broad guidelines. If they are not working for you, or you are concerned that you need further help taking it to the next level, get personalized help. There is no shame in asking questions.

When you try to explore different ways to improve your mind, body, and spiritual health, it shows perseverance to your wellness and sets an example for all. Through God, you are capable of far more than you will ever know.

Strategy three is to maintain. If you are happy with your health and you are at a comfortable level of activity that allows you to do the work you want to do to prevent disease and disability, then maintain your physical activity goals. It may be that you simply choose another walking route from the appendices in this book and study the corresponding biblical story to further your spiritual connection to physical activity. Give thanks that you are healthy and that God has given you many opportunities to use the strength you have obtained to do his work in the world.

When your physical health is about joyfully lifting up your capabilities to God, you will be happy. If you are obsessed with your physical health for your vanity, you will remain unhappy and unsatisfied. Our greatest joy comes from doing for others. When we make choices that are God-centered, we are filled with peace and contentment. God fills us with joy when we have set our hearts to a goal and become successful. God gave us food, drink, friends, and love to joyfully experience life and this fills our hearts. Living a healthy life is a godly life.

THOUGHTS TO PONDER

1. What was my daily average over the last thirty-six days for either steps or miles?

2. Where can I go from here?

3. For the next forty days, what will be my next goal?

This is what I have seen to be good: it is fitting to eat and drink and find enjoyment in all the toil with which one toils under the sun the few days of the life God gives us; for this is our lot. Likewise all to whom God gives wealth and possessions and whom he enables to enjoy them, and to accept their lot and find enjoyment in their toil—this is the gift of God. For they will scarcely brood over the days of their lives, because God keeps them occupied with the joy of their hearts. —Ecclesiastes 5:18–20

DAY 36   Steps taken: _____   Miles journeyed: _____

Exercise chosen: _____

Spiritual thoughts: _____

_____

_____

_____

Feelings: _____

_____

_____

_____

Motivating Your Church to Healthy Living

BIBLICAL BIG IDEA #37

"Do not work for food that perishes, but for food that endures for eternal life, which the Son of Man will give you. For it is on him that God the Father has set his seal." —John 6:27

When I first started Christ Walk I could not have done it without my church. While I wrote this book so that you could experience a Christ Walk outside of the church environment, it was ideally created to be a shared experience. I have run Christ Walk in some form for many years in small to medium to large group settings. I learned after the first year that the participants were far more successful in teams than on their own, and thus every time I do run a live Christ Walk there will always be teams formed as a part of the challenge. These little teams are little churches that pray together and form prayer teams to create a healthy physical and spiritual life for their group for the next forty days of the challenge. These teams go on to become pods of healthy living in their congregation.

Churches are essential not only for teaching people about healthy spiritual living, but also teaching people about healthy minds and bodies. Our churches are our communities of those with whom we share our lives. I want my church to be sensitive to the physical and dietary limitations of its members as it plans events. We *all* can stand to make healthier choices in our diets, not just the church member recovering from cancer or heart disease or diabetes. If we are all in this together, and faith heals, then our centers of healing and health should start at the church. If we are praying for health, longevity, and wellness for our church family, then we should also be acting as a healthy church family.

I have joked for years that the food eaten at church does not have calories. In truth, as I load up my plate at the smorgasbord of goodness (every church has a bevy of men and women who are wonderful cooks—it is hard to turn down any of their amazing creations), I am trying to allay my guilt at my overflowing plate. I can honestly say, though, that I do joyfully enjoy every morsel from church luncheons, breakfasts, and dinners even if there are calories involved. I love the table fellowship of Christians and the wonderful food. However, I am struck every time I attend a church meal that this is a wonderful opportunity to create healthy dinners, share the recipes, and nurture healthy choices and portion sizes among the members of this family. We may need to post on the church hall wall what a healthy portion looks like, or include the nutritional information on cards at the buffet, but we do have an opportunity to help each other make healthier choices.

As a family of believers in healthy living, we also have the opportunity to build Bible study and walking groups from the church and the larger community. If you host a weekly yoga and meditation event at your church, people will come. They will also become curious about what else the church has to offer and perhaps experience the love of God in new ways. If you host other athletic activities including youth sports and recreation, young families will come. If you host healthy cooking classes and dinners for young parents or families, they will come—probably along with some older, established families that are looking for inspiration in the kitchen!

At Emmanuel Church, we had a church member who loved to farm. His wife would say that she was the gardener and he was the farmer (I believe this was because she would weed and he would not). One year (prior to my attendance at the church) they received permission from a local business that had a large plot of unused land near the church to put in a community garden for all the church members. Members of the church either contributed a small amount of money towards seeds or seedlings they wanted to grow in the garden or provided the seeds themselves. Tom, the farmer, then sowed the seeds for the church and nurtured this garden into a massive fruit- and vegetable-producing bounty. Each Sunday he would place the offerings from the garden on a table in the church hall for anyone to take. Even if you did not provide seeds or money to the garden, there was more than enough bounty for all. After the church had taken their fill, the remainder would be taken to a local food shelter for use. The idea that a church can grow a community garden is an amazing idea. There is *nothing* healthier than fruits and vegetables directly from the ground. The work of the garden was the work of the church. Although Tom was the leader in the garden project, there were many other hands that helped to harvest and take care of the plot of land. It was an amazing gift to many individuals in the church who did not have the space at their homes or time in their lives to nurture a garden. And on top of that, the bounty fed not only the church, but the community as well. This little plot of garden was an amazing endeavor of "in-reach" and "out-reach" ministry that nurtured the health and physical wellness of the church, not only the spirit.

Every church has its group of runners. Challenge your runners to offer half marathon training groups for friends within the church who want to run but never have. Better yet, choose a ministry within or outside the church that your running team will commit to raising money for during their training period. Make running a part of the way your church does its mission business. And think about the amazing, healthy bodies that are being created by this endeavor. These strong bodies could be ready to help build the next Habitat for Humanity house, volunteer in the soup kitchen, or build a church or school in another country. These bodies will be strong to do the work of the church because the church has made a commitment to their bodies as well as their souls.

Many churches have forgotten how to nurture the mind and body and rely solely on preaching to the spirit. However, I know that the health of the individual is not just of the spirit; the entire mind, body, and spiritual connection needs to be nurtured.

I believe that things like community gardens, yoga exercises, meditation groups, and educational opportunities allow churches to nurture the physical and mental aspects of humanity while tying the message to the Holy Spirit.

[Paul says,]"So that you may lead lives worthy of the Lord, fully pleasing to him, as you bear fruit in every good work and as you grow in the knowledge of God. —Colossians 1:10

Exploring our knowledge of God through Christian education feeds our spirit; good nutrition, exercise, and healthy activities keeps our minds sharp and our bodies able to bear witness to the work God has called us to do as Christians. All these activities make for a healthier church. These activities reach out and call to the great community as a whole and provide opportunities to individuals without a church background to experience the love of God in many venues and not just the church pew. When we bring more people into the church, we provide them with the opportunity to feel the Holy Spirit and develop a life-long relationship with God. A church can be a new family to a person that has never had one. A church can be the avenue of opportunity to serve others and improve the lives of those around them near and far.

As a soon-to-be graduate of Christ Walk, you are the next seed in the garden of your church. It is your chance now to be a voice to healthy living and exploring opportunities for health in your church home. If you are shopping for a church, ask around until you find one that cares as much about your spirit as it does the temple that houses that spirit. It is all connected. As the seed in your church garden, suggest these ideas to your vestry or governing board of deacons (or however your church is set up to make decisions) and request more mind/body/spirit options.

Here are some considerations for building a healthy church:

- Start a Christ Walk group
- Host flow exercise and meditation classes
- Walk the labyrinth
- Start a community garden, and share the abundance not only in the church, but with the local soup kitchens/food banks
- Start a walking club
- Start a running club
- Host annual 5K run/walk events at the church—open to the community as a membership drive—tie to a local charity to raise money
- Make the annual picnic active with games and challenges for people of all ages
- Provide nutritional guidelines and visual representations of portion sizes during church meals
- Encourage your host of church cooks to explore healthier options that incorporate many fresh fruits and vegetables; challenge them to create an under-500-calorie meal that is delicious
- Ensure there is always a meatless option other than salad at a church meal
- Become a home for a Weight Watchers or other weight-loss group
- Begin a recycling program
- Explore great mission opportunities, including joining with other churches
- Challenge a neighboring church to a Christ Walk mileage challenge

- Host mind/body/spiritual Bible studies
- Host local medical or university experts on the health/spirit connection
- Provide fruits and vegetables, not just cookies and cake, at coffee hour
- Start a compost heap that church members can take from for garden fertilizers
- Strive to be a zero-waste church
- Host a yard sale
- Reestablish prayer groups that physically meet and pray
- Start a Facebook page/webpage that includes healthy tips and recipes
- Start a healthy recipe share group that goes out in the newsletter
- Feed not only the soul, but the body and mind
- Leverage your members of the nursing, medical, allied health professions to share their expertise
- Explore alternative medicine healing techniques
- Explore eating and cooking methods of the early church
- Host a Stations of the Cross fun run/walk
- Host a healing service
- Try something new

THOUGHTS TO PONDER

1. Is my church healthy?

2. What can I do to make it healthier?

3. Is there an idea from the above list that I would like to see happen at my church?

However that may be, let each of you lead the life that the Lord has assigned, to which God called you. This is my rule in all the churches. —1 Corinthians 7:17

DAY 37 Steps taken: _____ Miles journeyed: _____

Exercise chosen: _____

Spiritual thoughts: _____

_____

_____

_____

_____

Feelings: _____

_____

_____

_____

_____

DAY 38 Choices, Choices, Choices

BIBLICAL BIG IDEA #38

Now if you are unwilling to serve the LORD, choose this day whom you will serve, whether the gods your ancestors served in the region beyond the River or the gods of the Amorites in whose land you are living; but as for me and my household, we will serve the LORD."—Joshua 24:15

No matter the trials that your body throws at you, a state of health is obtainable. You *can* improve your health. I am passionate about health because health has been a real struggle for me my entire life. I am a little wary that, feeling like I have tackled my health trials, something new could be waiting around the corner. Thankfully, I have also learned that excess worry is not healthy, and I put these concerns in God's hands. I am doing what I can, with God's help. If anything else happens to me, I will tackle that too and move on, because I really do not believe my work in the world is done.

Healthy bodies are less likely to be subject to disease, illness, and injury. Does this mean that because you have an illness or injury or a disease or disability that you cannot make your body healthy within that context? No, on the contrary, it becomes *more* important to focus on improving your health. It will improve your management of the disease, and it can prevent further deterioration. While you may not be cured of your disease, you can be in a state of health and healing in the midst of your disease process. Curing and healing are two different things.

The choices I make in my daily life play a large role in how I manage my symptoms. When I choose to manage my autoimmune disease with lifestyle changes rather than drugs, I not only am able to control my symptoms, I am more aware of my body and how sensitive it is to my diet, environment, stress, and exercise choices. I am even more aware that many of the prescription drugs have impacted my health in the long term. I am now far more likely to look at means of managing my disease through what *I* can do, versus a short-term fix of a drug that has long-term impact on my wellbeing. These are my choices. Each of us has our own choices that are right for ourselves based on our own health.

Does this mean that I do not look with envy upon my husband, whose body does not seem to be affected by illness or disability? He seems to have a system that is stronger than mine, as viruses and colds roll off his shoulders. I, on the other hand, am sensitive to many things. I have come to learn that we are just made differently. Some people seem to have few problems, whereas others are simply plagued by one illness after another. Having a sensitive system, I have learned to value and prioritize my health greatly. It will always be important to me to take care of this temple because it is the only body I have.

There comes a point in many people's lives when they have to look at their health or the choices they are making and decide what is more important to them: their health or making poor choices. When I was losing my hearing, my first choice was either to stay on high-dose steroids (which at the time was the only thing besides methotrexate and IVIG infusions that seemed to stabilize the onslaught of the autoimmune process) and the damage it was wreaking on my body or take the gamble with losing my hearing. This is not to say that staying on these drugs would have prevented my hearing loss. Rather, it seemed as though it were simply slowing the process. If you have ever been on high-dose steroids, the effects are traumatic and long-lasting. I do not know what these drugs have done to my body in the long term. I was struggling; my body was not strong and full of health. I was looking at my body as though it would not be healthy if I was deaf. Instead, it was time to change my perception and look at what my body *could* do, even if deaf. So I got off all of the drugs, lost my hearing, and then God delivered cochlear implants. Six months after becoming completely deaf, I was the first child implanted at the Lahey Clinic in Boston, Massachusetts, with a cochlear implant. Twenty years later I heard out of my left ear for the first time by adding a second implant. When you change your perceptions, new doors and ideas of health will open to you.

Over the years, I have also been plagued with flare-ups of asthma, allergies, colitis, and other random autoimmune diseases. Usually, the doctors will put me on many drugs to control the flare-up. Usually, I feel a lot worse from the medications than the disease. I have found that making changes to my lifestyle and the healthy choices I make can be as effective, or more so, than the medications the doctor may have prescribed. This is not to say that traditional medicine is not an effective means for treating illnesses. On the contrary, making changes to your lifestyle will go hand in hand with any approach identified with your health care provider. As I have read more and become wiser about my body, I have learned to control these flare-ups by changing my environment and focusing on organic eating and clean living. By making healthier choices in my diet, I was able to get off of years of medications and have never had a problem with colitis since. In the last year, I was told that I had rheumatoid arthritis and would need to go on methotrexate for treatment. After my experience with my hearing loss, this broke me into a cold sweat! Instead, I chose to research alternatives to drug therapy, and again cleaned out my pantry. (I seem to get a little more organic and a little cleaner in my diet each time something like this happens because I realize that what I put in my mouth does make a difference.) I started acupuncture, and have remained drug-free without pain, inflammation, or drugs. These were my choices. The choices you make for addressing your health should be done in concert with your healthcare provider and should include research into the changes you can make in your lifestyle to complement your disease management plan.

You may not choose an Eastern approach to managing disease like I did, but I want you to be aware that you have choices with your health. There are always alternatives to how we treat our bodies. Good food can be healing. Good nutrition is the first line of defense in disease. What we put in our bodies and what we do with them (exercise or lack thereof) make a huge impact in how we manage disease or how our body responds to treatment. We can start making choices to have healthier bodies if we make health our priority. These choices are a lifelong commitment, not just for forty days or until we have reached a certain goal. Obtaining and maintaining health is a choice we make every day. Sometimes we do not make the best choices, but the good thing is that the next time we do make a choice we always have the option to make a new healthy choice.

Why do I talk about choice so much? I believe we all have choices. Our Christian life is a choice. It is only *you* that can control *you*. I know that when people try to change it takes many failures and many attempts before reaching a successful change. It also takes many repetitions of the behavior to become the norm. This is a choice that only you can make for you. God will help you through those choices if you let God be a part of not only your spiritual health but also your physical health.

A lifetime of health is less of a burden on our friends and families. A strong body is one with fewer struggles. A healthy temple is one that is primed to hear God's call for action in the world instead of being focused on everything that is wrong with it. No matter the state of your body, it is here to do God's work in the world. No matter the state of health you have, you can always make healthier choices to make that body stronger. It is your choice.

THOUGHTS TO PONDER

1. Am I feeling that my body is stronger after these forty days?

2. If not, what do I need to do?

3. Do I feel that my lifestyle changes have been made more in tune with my body's needs or improved my health? If so, way to go!!

Finally, brothers and sisters, we ask and urge you in the Lord Jesus that, as you learned from us how you ought to live and to please God (as, in fact, you are doing), you should do so more and more. —1 Thessalonians 4:1

DAY 38 Steps taken: _____ Miles journeyed: _____

Exercise chosen: _____

Spiritual thoughts: _____

_____

_____

_____

Feelings: _____

_____

_____

_____

God's Grace

BIBLICAL BIG IDEA #39

With great power the apostles gave their testimony to the resurrection of the Lord Jesus, and great grace was upon them all. —Acts 4:33

God's grace is amazing. I am awed by the journey that God has guided us on over the last thirty-nine days. God has been with us every step of the way. God is at work in each of us. As I have reiterated over and over, we are on earth for God's mission. We have a purpose here and God's grace guides us on that mission.

God's grace can transform our bodies if we are partners with God on the journey ahead. When God gave us freedom of choice to make our own decisions, it was up to us to make the changes in our bodies that are needed. God's grace gives us the strength to make those changes. It is also up to us to take up the charge of God's work in the world and be an emissary of God's love.

God's grace overcomes fear of these changes. When I find fear overwhelming, it fills me with anxiety and trepidation for the future. Through prayer, I open a gateway to God's grace that washes away my fears and anxiety.

The early Christians led a structured life centered on prayer, fasting, worship, and activity that was done to the glory of God. When we want to make changes in ourselves to a more Christ-centered life, it is imperative that we develop this same discipline. If we take the time for Christian practices, then we are building an ordered life that allows God's grace to be a part of every day of our lives. I build my discipline through scheduling. This sets a tempo for how I ensure that mind, body, and spiritual health are a part of every moment in my life. I have a very type-A personality, so scheduling ensures that I have made time for the priorities that are important to me:

5:00 a.m.: Wake

5:15 a.m.: Coffee, tea, prayer, meditation

5:30–6:30 a.m.: Exercise

6:30–8:00 a.m.: Kids and school

8:00 a.m.–12:00 p.m.: Work

12:00–1:00 p.m.: Lunch and prayer

1:00–3:00 p.m.: Work

3:00–5:00 p.m.: Kids, activities

5:00–6:00 p.m.: Dinner prep and homework

6:00–7:00 p.m.: Dinner and prayer

7:00–8:00 p.m.: Bath

8:00 p.m.: Bedtime for kids

8:00–10:00 p.m.: Time with spouse

10:00 p.m.: Bedtime and prayers

This is an example of one of my schedules. In truth, my schedule varies around the time of the year, what is going on in life, and how things crop up. I do find that no matter the variance in my schedule, HAVING a schedule helps keep my priorities in order.

Because prayer is included at intervals throughout the day, Christ is a part of everything that I do. With Christ at my side through my daily life, I have a pulse check on what is important and what is not. When God does not feel close to me in my life, I know it is I who have strayed and not God. God's grace is ever present for me to weave it back in my life. I am far more content when I remember to include God in my schedule, than not.

Through this journey in Christ Walk, God's grace has been with us. As we go on from Christ Walk, we will need to focus on how to continue to include God as a part of our call towards mind, body, and spiritual health. God has been with us as we discussed and discovered prayer. God has been with us as we pondered physical fitness and healing. God has been with us as we prayed for spiritual growth and transformation.

God has been with me as I wrote this book. At times, I have heard God's voice more clearly than at others, and I apologize for those moments when the message has not been clear. Having come to this point, I hope you have been transformed as well. I believe that you can be changed. If you have not felt God's grace in your life these past forty days, I pray that, in time, you will pick this book up and try again. God's grace is available at any time and any place we need it. We need simply to ask. We can be made new through the Holy Spirit, allowing God's grace to work through us. We are nothing without God.

THOUGHTS TO PONDER

1. Do I feel God's grace in my life?

2. How can I open myself up to the power of God's grace?

3. What is God's grace calling me to do next on my journey?

But I do not count my life of any value to myself, if only I may finish my course and the ministry that I received from the Lord Jesus, to testify to the good news of God's grace. —Acts 20:24

DAY 39 Steps taken: _____ Miles journeyed: _____

Exercise chosen: _____

Spiritual thoughts: _____

_____

_____

_____

Feelings: _____

_____

_____

_____

Where Do I Go
from Here?

BIBLICAL BIG IDEA #40

*I thank my God every time I remember you, constantly praying
with joy in every one of my prayers for all of you, because of
your sharing in the gospel from the first day until now. I am
confident of this, that the one who began a good work among
you will bring it to completion by the day of Jesus Christ.*
—Philippians 1:3–6

I hope by this point in Christ Walk you realize that this is not the end
of the journey. This was just one forty-day period of your life. There are
many more days to lead a Christ Walk way of life—body, mind, and soul.
I hope you feel renewed, redeemed, and rejuvenated to make each day
and each choice you make as healthy as possible. Each choice should be
a proclamation of health to the glory of God. You are God's temple. You
are God's emissary into the world and the healthy face you present to the
world should be a beacon for others to live a healthy life, too. If you have
done Christ Walk as a part of a Lenten discipline, it is now Easter. We
have been resurrected through Christ to a life eternal. Consider your way
forth as a rebirth in healthy living!

If you made changes in your life these past forty days—way to go!
Keep up the good work and do not stop your good works in your life.
If not, that is all right as well. Through the grace of God, we have every
chance to try again.

*They are now justified by his grace as a gift, through the redemption that is in
Christ Jesus.* —Romans 3:24

We all have a chance to make a difference because we are all redeemed
through Christ to do so. God gives us many chances. I prayerfully hope
that you continue the Christ Walk journey the remainder of your life.
Forty days is a powerful period in the Bible. There are many "forty days"

in your life to be transformed and allow God's grace to do amazing things through you.

You have made changes in your life the last forty days (I hope!). Perhaps you have made leaps and bounds in your personal health. Does this mean you will not have to ever worry about your health again? Does this mean you will not face health challenges? Unfortunately, I cannot predict that. You have reduced your risk, but life happens.

Then Hezekiah said to Isaiah, "The word of the LORD that you have spoken is good." For he thought, "Why not, if there will be peace and security in my days?" —2 Kings 20:19

Hezekiah wondered if there would ever be a time when he did not have to worry. Would he ever be able to sit back and rest on his laurels? The bottom line is no. We never stop working on our relationship with God, we never stop taking care of our temples and preparing ourselves for everlasting life with God.

No one knows what the world has in store for you. Through prayer, you will hear what God has planned for you, but remember we do not know what we have been exposed to, or what could change our bodies, or impact our health in the long term. We must put this in God's hands and realize that even with this masterful, healthy temple we have built, tragedy may befall it. Through God, we will get through this as well. Through God, any temple can be rebuilt and repurposed. We go from here with the grace of God to continue this journey, to be vigilant, and to keep trying. While we are redeemed by God's grace, that does not preclude us from trying and trying again.

For it is God who is at work in you, enabling you both to will and to work for his good pleasure. —Philippians 2:13

There is a reason for you here on this earth. There is a reason for you to be healthy and there is a reason for you to continue to take care of yourself mind, body, and spirit. Your temple is taking God's spark out into the world. Keep it walking.

God's grace to you as you continue your journey. It has been an honor to share myself with you these last forty days and I prayerfully hope that you will keep Christ Walking.

Peace. Enjoy every moment of the journey and remember that Christ is with you every step of the way.

~*Anna*

DAY 40 Steps taken: _____ Miles journeyed: _____

Exercise chosen: _____

Spiritual thoughts: _____

_____

_____

_____

_____

Feelings: _____

_____

_____

_____

_____

PULSE CHECK REDEMPTION

We are only redeemed through God. It is God's grace that helps us to make changes in our life. Through the last forty days, we have used Christ Walk to change our bodies and nourish our souls and minds. God's redemption is amazing. It can change us in ways we never imagined. Following God is life-changing and life-inspiring. No matter what we have done, to ourselves or others, we can be changed by the spirit of God. Christ Walk has allowed God to journey with us as we work to change ourselves—body, mind, and spirit. We can be made new, made whole, and created for God's purpose once again.

He sent redemption to his people; he has commanded his covenant forever. Holy and awesome is his name. —Psalm 111:9

O Israel, hope in the LORD! For with the LORD there is steadfast love, and with him is great power to redeem. —Psalm 130:7

God loves us without fail. God's covenant with us does not waver and is always available to us. God will be ready to receive our repentance when we find ourselves falling into sin again with our body, mind, or soul.

They are now justified by his grace as a gift, through the redemption that is in Christ Jesus. —Romans 3:24

We are not redeemed by anything we do; we are redeemed through God. Our acts of repentance show God that we are ready to see the redemption that was always there. We can choose to have a relationship with God whenever we want. We are transformed by Christ's living sacrifice for us. Christ Walk is an opportunity to redeem our bodies from a life of poor choices and to redeem that body to Christ's work in the world. When we are doing Christ's work in the world, we are showing God's love to others. The more we walk on the Christ Walk path, the more we open ourselves up to God's love and redemption.

Christ Walk always.

Appendices

APPENDIX A
Suggested Walking Routes*

Individual and Beginner Routes

Name of Route	Description	Total Distance	Distance Per Day
Nazareth Challenge	The route between Jesus' hometown of Nazareth and Jerusalem	65 miles	1.6 miles or 4,000 steps per day
Jerusalem to Damascus	Paul's conversion on the Damascus Road took place along this journey.	150 miles	3.75 miles or 7,500 steps per day

Intermediate Routes

Name of Route	Description	Total Distance	Distance Per Day
The Jerusalem Challenge	The *Via Dolorosa* (Way of Sorrows) is the route Jesus took through Jerusalem during the last week of his life, which included his preaching in the Temple, clearing the Temple of the money-changers, his Last Supper with the disciples, his arrest in the Garden of Gethsemane, his trial, and his crucifixion.	88 miles	2.2 miles or about 5,500 steps per day
Damascus to Caesarea	One of Paul's missionary journeys	200 miles	5 miles or 10,000 steps per day (a pedometer is recommended)

*All distances are approximate and renditions from maps of the Holy Land.

Advanced

Name of Route	Description	Total Distance	Distance Per Day
The Bethlehem Challenge	The distance between Bethlehem and Jerusalem, representing the beginning and end of Christ's life	200 miles	5 miles or 10,000 steps per day (without using a pedometer)*

*This challenge is done without a pedometer. This means that you will get 5 miles of exercise during one workout instead of accumulating the miles over the course of a day with a pedometer.

Name of Route	Description	Total Distance	Distance Per Day
Tarsus to Jerusalem Challenge	One of Paul's missionary journeys	390 miles	9.75 miles of 19,500 steps per day (pedometer recommended)
The Exodus Challenge	The route the Israelites traveled to get to the Promised Land of Canaan	375 miles	9.4 miles or 18,750 steps per day (pedometer recommended)

Group Challenges

Pool each individual participant's miles each week to reach a group distance goal.

Name of Route	Description	Total Distance	Distance Per Day
The Abraham Migration	Represents Abraham's wanderings to find the Promised Land to begin the birth of God's people	900 miles	22.5 miles per day
Jerusalem to Antioch (round trip)	One of Paul's missionary journeys	705 miles	17.25 miles per day
Paul's First Missionary Journey	Paul's first mission trip	1,300 miles	32.5 miles per day
Ephesus to Jerusalem	One of Paul's missionary trips	800 miles	20 miles per day
Jerusalem to Rome	The end of the road for Paul	1,800 miles	45 miles per day

Group Challenges (continued)

Name of Route	Description	Total Distance	Distance Per Day
Jerusalem to Corinth	One of Paul's missionary journeys	1,050 miles	26.25 miles per day
Antioch to Philippi	A portion of Paul's third missionary journey	950 miles	23.75 miles per day

Beginner Walks

Nazareth Challenge: It is 65 miles between Jesus' hometown of Nazareth and Jerusalem. This is approximately 1.6 miles each day for forty days to walk the distance of the route that Jesus preached to reach his end in Jerusalem. Set a goal to walk 1.6 miles each day or 4,000 steps per day during Lent (or any forty day period of your choosing), or complete 65 miles by the end of the six-week period.

Jerusalem to Damascus: This journey represents Paul's conversion on the Damascus Road. It is 150 miles or 3.75 miles per day or 7,500 steps a day.

Intermediate Walks

Jerusalem Challenge: During Jesus' final days, his route through Jerusalem included preaching at the Temple, clearing the Temple of the money changers, the last supper with his disciples, his arrest in the Garden of Gethsemane, his trial, Peter's denial, and his crucifixion. This route was approximately 2.2 miles in length. Set a goal to walk 2.2 miles each day during Lent, or about 5,500 steps per day.

Damascus to Caesarea: One of Paul's missionary journeys was about 200 miles or 5 miles per day or 10,000 steps a day. You can use a pedometer throughout the day to accumulate the miles.

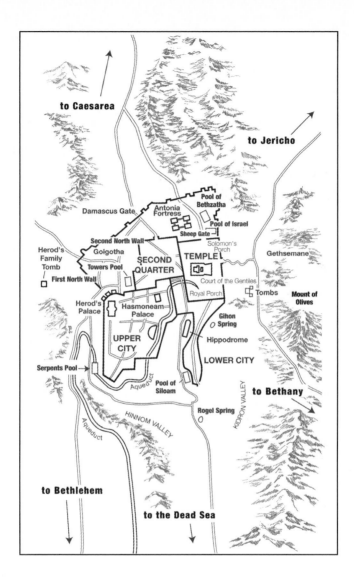

Advanced Walks

Bethlehem Challenge: It is five miles between Bethlehem and Jerusalem. This represents the beginning to the end of Christ's journey. Set a goal to walk five miles without using a pedometer.

Tarsus to Jerusalem: This is Paul's route from his home town of Tarsus to Jerusalem. I look at this journey as a reflection of where we started in life and what draws us on our calling with Christ. 390 miles or 9.75 miles a day or 19,500 steps a day

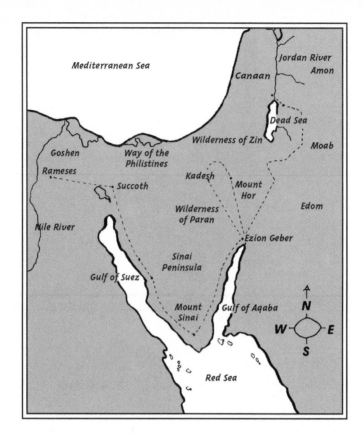

The Exodus: The route the Israelites traveled to get to the Promised Land is 375 miles, 9.4 miles per day or 18,750 steps per day. (This may be used as a group challenge.)

Group Challenges

These goals should be divided based on the number of people in your group and how many miles each group member will commit to walking during the forty-day challenge:

The Abraham Migration: This represents Abraham's wanderings to find the Promised Land to begin the birth of God's people. It is roughly 900 miles, or 22.5 miles a day.

Jerusalem to Antioch: This is the first part of Paul's second missionary journey. Paul was preaching to the Gentiles in Antioch. This was one of the first times in which God's word was shared to other Christians not of Jewish descent. This is a round trip of 705 miles or 17.25 miles a day.

Antioch to Cyprus: This is part of Paul's 1st missionary journey. Paul and Barnabas travel from Antioch to Barnabas' home in Salamis, Cyprus to preach the word of God. 1,300 miles or 32.5 miles a day

Ephesus to Jerusalem: This is a portion of Paul's third missionary journey. The Letter to the Ephesians is one of Paul's most famous letters written while building the church in the city of Ephesus. The church later became one of the heads of the seven churches of Asia Minor and contributed to the spread of Christianity across what is modern day Turkey. 800 miles or 20 miles a day

Paul's Journey to Rome: Paul's journey from Jerusalem to Rome where he finally died for his beliefs. It is said that Paul's body is buried underneath St. Paul's Cathedral in Vatican City. 1,800 miles or 45 miles a day

Jerusalem to Corinth: The full route of Paul's third missionary journey to Corinth, Greece. Paul is the founder of the Christian church in Corinth. In his letter to the Corinthians, Paul gives thanks for his health, his journey, his deliverance from dangers, and for the people of Corinth. 1050 miles or 26.25 miles a day

Antioch to Philippi: This is a portion of Paul's 3rd Missionary Journey. The church in Philippi is the first Christian church founded by Paul in Europe. 950 miles or 23.75 miles a day

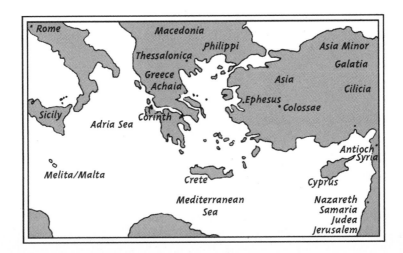

Pedometer Usage and Mileage Calculations

You can purchase a pedometer from any sporting or general goods store. When you clip your pedometer onto your waistband, it should be at about the height of your hipbone. Roughly 2,000 steps equal a mile, but steps and mileage calculation depend on the length of your stride. For the ease of calculation you can use 2,000 steps to a mile, or measure your stride and have the pedometer calculate it for you. You do not have to walk; you can use a treadmill, run, bike, swim or whatever activity you choose to do. Approximately fifteen minutes of physical activity will equal a mile if you are unable to calculate the mileage. (For example, fifteen minutes of an aerobics/yoga class would be a mile for the purpose of this program.)

If you are unable to exercise, consider using each fifteen-minute block in volunteering or in prayer. Our goal is to transform spiritually as well as physically. There are no penalties in Christ Walk! Focus on things you can do to change your life through increased activity, or increased prayer, or increased work for others. Use your pedometer all day so that *all* of your activity will be included towards your goal. Please join us in a journey taking a step of faith in Christ.

Mileage Calculation Chart

Activity	Time	Steps	Record Miles As:
Walking	15–20 minutes	2,000–2,500	1 or distance on route
Running	Varies	2,000–2,500	Check route distance
Biking	Varies	N/A	Check odometer distance
Aerobics	15 minutes	Varies	1
Dancing	15 minutes	Varies	1
Yoga	15 minutes	Varies	1
Prayer/Meditation	15 minutes	Varies	1
Volunteerism	15 minutes	Varies	1

A Few Healthy Eating and Exercise Habits

HEALTHY EATING

- Eat slowly and at a table
- Limit distractions like TV, phone, news (*This allows you to enjoy the food you're eating and makes you more aware of what you're eating.*)
- Eat regular meals and plan snacks (*This allows you to stay in control of eating and increases metabolic rate.*)
- Exercise three to five times a week
- Enjoy eating
- Relax and slow down (*It takes twenty minutes for the brain to know you are full. Eating fast leads to excessive eating.*)
- Drink liquids between bites
- Set down utensils (spoon/chopsticks)
- Chew and savor food while you eat
- *Enjoy* sharing meal time

TIPS TO SPEED UP YOUR METABOLISM

- Quit starving yourself
- Start exercising
- Exercise longer
- Exercise large muscle groups
- Vary your workout

SETTING REALISTIC EXERCISE GOALS

- Walk to work
- Exercise (sit-ups, push-ups, jumping jacks, etc.) in front of the TV
- Walk during lunch hour
- Walk instead of driving whenever you can
- Take a family walk after dinner
- Mow your lawn with a push mower
- Walk to your place of worship instead of driving
- Walk your kids to school
- Join an exercise group
- Replace Sunday drive with Sunday walk

SUPPORTING YOUR GOALS

- For the most part, we control our environment
- Are you taking extra steps every day to increase physical activity in your life?
- Are you making healthy choices?
- It's not about punishment and denial, it's about good choices
- Change is difficult, even if it's about small choices
- Consistency: The #1 key to success
  - The more you exercise, the easier it gets
  - When all else fails, keep going
  - The more frequently you make healthy food choices, the easier it gets

OTHER STICK-TO STRATEGIES

- Use a pedometer
- Christ Walk!
- Get a dog!
- Leave yourself exercise reminders like setting your walking shoes out for your morning walk before you go to bed
- Clean your pantry of temptations! (Would you keep the devil in your back pocket?)
- Make sure you are having fun with whatever you choose to do!

APPENDIX D

Suggestions for Groups

Christ Walk was intended to be a group activity. People who have communities of fitness or teams of fitness are more likely to be successful in their goals. Teams are successful when they:

- Meet together
- Exercise together
- Pray together
- Share successes and challenges together
- Encourage each other

If you are not experiencing Christ Walk as a part of a church educational or devotional period, try to get a group of friends together to experience the lessons and activities together. Your Bible study, men's, or women's group can complete Christ Walk. The purpose is to commit to improving your health together as you help each other along to a healthier you. If you do not have access to a group, join a virtual team through Fitbit, Facebook, or other group so that you are not alone in your journey.

Christ Walk can be found online at:

- Facebook: www.facebook.com/christwalk40day
- Twitter: @christwalk1
- Blog: www.blogspot.christwalk40day.com

Another suggestion for groups is to invite a fitness professional to discuss principles of fitness as a special guest. I also recommend a fitness professional come to conduct fitness testing with each individual followed by individualized fitness plan recommendations based on the results of the fitness test for everyone.

APPENDIX E

Ideas for a Youth Christ Walk Group

Find someone in your group you don't know and introduce yourself, telling them something unique about you. Keep talking and asking questions until you figure out what you have in common. Once you know what you have in common, find a group of two and repeat the exercise until the four have something in common. Repeat this process until the group is complete and the whole group has discovered something that they have in common. (It cannot be church or Christ Walk!)

When the ice breaker is complete, you can then work as a group to come up with:

- A team name

- A team prayer—write it as a group

- Your team's walking/mileage goal

- Your individual walking/running/biking/etc. goal

Brainstorm something that you would like to raise money for by completing that goal (a mission you would like to support) and how to do it. Consider finding a fun walk/run to do together as a team towards the end of Lent—not mandatory, just an idea for fundraising. People could sponsor you or your team a dollar per mile, or something for completing the race, or completing your mileage journey.

Suggestions for Group Leaders

If you are taking on the role as a Christ Walk group leader, congratulations! What an awesome experience for you and your team or church. You can join the Christ Walk forum on Facebook to discuss ideas and goals with members of the Christ Walk community around the globe! I am happy to provide feedback or guidance on running a group Christ Walk. Christ Walk can be found online at:

- Facebook: www.facebook.com/christwalk40day
- Twitter: @christwalk1
- Blog: www.blogspot.christwalk40day.com

The number one guidance I offer in leading Christ Walk is to give freely of yourself and your experience. You may have a lot of fitness experience or none at all, but since we all have health, we all have a perspective that can be shared and discussed in our small-group settings that are valuable to anyone in the room. I have led groups from as few as five participants to as many as eighty, and the experience can be as much as we choose to share with each other during our time together. Give freely of yourself and your experience. This builds a bond of a shared experience.

There are several ways that the Christ Walk experience can be structured for groups:

- As a simple Bible study, meet each week to discuss the "Thoughts to Ponder" after each day's reading. Simply share your experiences with those meditations. Make sure that everyone reports and tracks their miles to their destination.
- Meet each week to focus on a different topic (See Appendix G for an outline):
  - Week One: Introduction
  - Week Two: Physical Health

- ○ Week Three: Mental Health
- ○ Week Four: Spiritual Health
- ○ Week Five: Nutrition
- ○ Week Six: Pot Luck and Graduation/Sharing
- Meet each week to discuss one of the scripture readings from the meditations, sharing what each says to the members of your group about their health.
  - ○ Week One: Introduction
  - ○ Week Two: Yoga
  - ○ Week Three: Aerobics
  - ○ Week Four: Guided Walk
  - ○ Week Five: Weight Lifting
  - ○ Week Six: Meditation
- Meet each week and have a theological reflection on one of the topics on the week's readings. Discuss the topic from the point of view of creation, sin, judgment, repentance, and redemption. (See Appendix G for an outline.)
  - ○ Week One: Introduction
  - ○ Week Two: Creation—How is God creating something new in us?
  - ○ Week Three: Sin—Where have we gone wrong?
  - ○ Week Four: Judgment—Where are we caught up short?
  - ○ Week Five: Repentance—Where have we sought forgiveness?
  - ○ Week Six: Redemption—Where have we been forgiven?
- Meet each week and provide keys to healthy living.
  - ○ Week One: Introduction
  - ○ Week Two: Health Fair/Health Assessment
  - ○ Week Three: Making Change/Change Exercise/Goal Setting
  - ○ Week Four: Fitness Testing
  - ○ Week Five: Cooking Classes
  - ○ Week Six: Healthy Potluck

Need other Ideas? Join me on Facebook, Twitter, or the blog for a discussion of group options. I am happy to answer questions as they are posted!

Happy Christ Walking!

Christ Walk Program Outlines

Christ Walk makes a perfect program for adults (or youth) who desire to improve or change their habits toward a healthier life—body, mind, and spirit. Each week correlates to a section of *Christ Walk* (the book), and each participant should have a copy for recording their progress in the journal sections.

Options

- Day or evening sessions: 1 hour
- Evenings with a meal and worship: 2.5 hours
  - Pot Luck meal—1 hour
  - Session—1 hour
  - Compline or Evening Prayer—30 minutes
- Session with a meal: 2 hours
  - Potluck meal—1 hour
  - Session—1 hour

Two models are offered here for holding your own Christ Walk program in your church, organization, or with friends. Feel free to mix them together, substitute your own activities, or adapt to create your own program. Consider offering childcare during the sessions, or holding a children's program concurrent with the adult program. It is never too early to help our children build healthy habits for body, mind, and spirit!

Useful Materials

It is useful to have a number of materials available for the class meeting times. A list of tools I have on hand when I lead a Christ Walk group include:

- A computer and projector with any PowerPoint presentations you may use to help with the weekly discussions
- Poster board or newsprint (with markers) for the teams to use for the activity
- Newsprint, easel, and tape for the leader to write up brainstorming comments and important discussion points
- A poster of all the team names and routes chosen (You can have them add up their miles each week and put it on their team poster.)

Publicity

When organizing a class, make sure to spread the word using your church's newsletter, weekly bulletin, website, Facebook page, or even the local newspaper. Here are two samples you can adapt.

Newsletter article sample #1

Have you ever wondered what it would have been like to walk with Jesus? There were no cars two thousand years ago. Jesus walked throughout his ministry. The "Christ Walk" program allows us to walk the miles of various routes in the Bible during the next forty days. Walking is a very holy activity that almost anyone can do at any fitness level. The benefits of walking are numerous for every age. Some of the routes that we can explore include the *Via Dolorosa* (Christ's last walk through Jerusalem), the Nazareth-Jerusalem route, Paul's missionary journeys, the spread of Christianity from Jerusalem to Rome, and many more. I invite you to join us on a journey of a lifetime as we study mind, body, and spiritual health with "Christ Walk: A 40-Day Spiritual Fitness Program."

The Christ Walk program will be offered at (*insert your church/address*) beginning on (*insert dates and times*) as a forty-day mind, body and spiritual wellness program for Lent (*or any other season or timeframe*). Individuals and teams will select various routes of the Bible and count steps or miles towards their goal. Each week we will meet in fellowship to have a program on a different aspect of mind, body, and spiritual health. Teams will participate in reflective exercises that will help them grow towards a Christ-centered life. Every aspect of what we do can be lifted as an offering to God, even taking care of our bodies. There is a "God-spark" in each of us and our bodies are the temple that God gives us to explore our gifts and talents. Taking care of that body to do God's work is paramount.

If you are interested in Christ Walk, or would like more information on the program, please contact (*insert contact information*). Christ Walk is available to anyone at any fitness level. A participant even walked her routes with her walker! You can experience Christ Walk, too. Peace and happy trails, (*your name*).

Newsletter article sample #2

An amazing thing will happen this Lent (*or other forty-day/6 week period*) at church! We will get to exercise and eat at the same time! Study Suppers return with various groups within the church catering a lovely dinner of soup and salad each Wednesday (*or other day*) at 6:00 p.m. in the Parish Hall. Dinner will be followed by the Christ Walk program, a forty-day walking program than encompasses mind, body, and spiritual health during the forty days of Lent.

- Week 1: Introduction and goal-setting
- Week 2: (insert topic)
- Week 3: (insert topic)
- Week 4: (insert topic)
- Week 5: (insert topic)
- Week 6: Healthy potluck and graduation (optional)

Childcare will be available and there will be a special youth team option. Join us starting (*insert date*) at (*insert time*) in the Parish Hall. There will be a sign-up sheet in the church so that we can ensure there are enough materials for everyone interested in participating. The program is open to all, no matter your health or fitness level. If you have questions, feel free to contact (*insert contact name*) via (*email*) or (*phone*). See you on the journey!

Ice Breakers

ICE BREAKER A: INTRODUCE A NEW FRIEND

- Pair up with someone you do not know
- Ask them to take one to three things from their wallet, purse, pocket, etc., and use those three things to describe themselves
- Introduce your partner to the group

ICE BREAKER B: FORMING TEAMS

- Pair up with someone you do not know
- Ask each other questions until you find something you have in common
- Go find another team you do not know—talk to each other until you find something all four of you have in common
- Do this one more time until you have a group of six (or four to five, depending on group totals: You are building your walking teams with this method.)
- Choose a group speaker who tells the larger group what you all have in common
- Look closely at the people in your group
- This is your Christ Walk team!
- Pray for each other!

ICE BREAKER C: BIBLE STUDY

This can also serve as the introduction to the program as you move into the leader discussion points.

- "And this is love, that we walk according to his commandments; this is the commandment just as you have heard from the beginning—you must walk in it." 2 John 1:6
- What does walking in love mean? Discuss in small groups.
- Share with the larger group
- Leader points that can be shared:
  - We are called to walk with Christ in our everyday life
  - We can use the Holy Spirit to work towards better mind, body, and spiritual health
  - We walk to do God's work
  - We walk to make our bodies stronger to do God's work
  - We pray to do God's work
  - Our mind, body, and spiritual health are for us to do God's work
  - Christ Walk is. . . the journey of making our bodies stronger, mind, body, and spirit, to DO God's work for all of our lives

Example 1
Walking with Christ: A Five or Six-Week Program

Week 1: Introducing Christ Walk

Week 2: Christ Calls Us to Change

Week 3: What is Health? A Group Reflection on the Definition of Health

Week 4: Meditation and Health *or* Nutrition and Health

Week 5: Where Do I Go From Here? Keeping the Journey Going

Week 6: Healthy Potluck (optional)

Week 1: Introducing Christ Walk
Gather

Open with Prayer
You can assign weekly prayer duties to each of the teams in your group if you have a large enough group, or ask volunteers to lead opening and closing prayer each week.

Introduce an Ice Breaker

Presentation and Discussion

Leader's Talking Points
- We are called to walk with Christ in our everyday life
- Mind, body, and spirit
- Each day we should resolve to walk with Christ
- "This is the day that the Lord has made, let us rejoice and be glad in it."
- We can use the Holy Spirit to work towards better mind, body, and spiritual health

We'll be using the actual motion of "walking with Christ" during this challenge and goal towards better mind, body, and spiritual health. This goal will be a metaphor for many changes in our lives and how we are called to serve Christ, how we stick with it, how we might slip up, and how we take this on to the rest of our lives.

- With this challenge you begin your commitment to walk with Christ.

- You will choose a walking challenge to work on during Lent (or whatever time frame you have chosen).
- You can choose to pair up with a buddy to work together towards your walk with Christ.
- You will choose an individual goal and your group will choose a group goal. (This is a good time to distribute the Christ Walk books and check out the appendices.)
- There is room in the back of your book to track your daily miles towards your goal.
- Each day in your book includes journal space to help you on your way:
  - Spaces to record distance
  - Spaces to record reflective thoughts on journey
  - Daily prayers and thoughts on a Christ-centered life

Considerations for Walking

- You may use a pedometer (step counter) to measure your distance each day. Approximately 2,000 to 2,500 steps equals 1 mile. (Option: Distribute pedometers to each participant.)
- You do not have to walk; you can use a treadmill, run, bike, swim, or whatever activity you can measure in terms of miles.
- If you cannot measure mileage, roughly fifteen minutes of physical activity (like an aerobics class) equals one mile. The important thing is to choose something to be physically active.
- Document miles in mile tracker in Christ Walk—there is a table in the back of the book to use *(see page 220)*.
- If you get a pedometer or a Fitbit or other fitness-tracking device, (available at places like Target, Wal-Mart or any other sporting goods store), we can discuss use at the next class. Otherwise, start keeping track of the steps and miles you are taking with your new fitness tracker.

Activity: Your Walking Team

- Break into team(s)
- Brainstorm team name
- Develop short team prayer
- Agree on team walking goal
- Share with the larger group

Conclusion

Wrap-Up

- Review mind, body, and spiritual journey
- Develop a Christ-centered life through mind, body, and spiritual exercises (exercise, study, eat good food, pray and/or meditate!)
- Questions?

Homework

- Choose a walking challenge
- Meditate on the purpose of your goal and the change you want to happen in the next six weeks
- Purchase pedometer, or Fitbit, or other fitness tracker
- Pray for your team

Close with Prayer

Week 2: Christ Calls Us to Change

Gather

Open with Prayer

Presentation and Discussion

Leader's Talking Points

- We've committed to a mind, body, and spiritual journey towards total well being
- You have begun your physical walk with Christ
- Let's discuss how Christ calls us to change our lives to be more Christ-centered
- Discuss the Change Exercise (below) and the three most important things in your life from Day 5 of "Christ Walk"

Activity: "Christ Calls Us to Change" Exercise
Distribute paper and pencils to each participant. Directions:

- Write your name
- Write the most important things in your life under your name
- Turn the piece of paper over and write one thing that you would like to change or work on during Lent (or whatever time frame you are following)

- How does the thing you want to change about yourself reflect on what you say are the most important things in your life?

- Is God one of the most important things in your life?

- How does your habit reflect on your relationship with God?

- Can you use your relationship with God to help you work on what you want to change?

Open the floor to discussion or questions. Ask if anyone wants to share his or her own personal goal to change. Volunteer what you want to change about yourself. Give freely of your experience.

Let's brainstorm how we can use God to work on mind, body, and spiritual wellbeing to help us change. Note these on newsprint.

Goal Discussion:
Leader's Talking Points:

- Giving up chocolate, caffeine, alcohol, sweets, meat, etc.

- Taking on readings, mission work, prayer

- Results in self-discipline and spiritual discipline especially if you use prayer and the Holy Spirit as your source of strength towards giving up indulgences

Conclusion

Wrap-Up

- What did you decide you wanted to change for this challenge?

- What are some tools that you have to support you through this?

- Do the three most important things in your life support what you want to change?

- If not, do you need to rethink the most important things in your life?

- Questions? Thoughts?

Close with Prayer

Week 3: Group Discussion: What is Health?

Gather

Open with Prayer

Presentation and Discussion

Leader's Talking Points

Taking care of our body is like taking care of Christ as we are made in his image. A whole and healthy body is a body that can be more devoted to his call in your life.

The World Health Organization's definition of health: "Health is a state of complete physical, mental, and social wellbeing and not merely the absence of disease or infirmity."

Activity: What Does Health Look Like?

Leader's Talking Points:

Print the above definition on newsprint and record your conversation on the following for all to see:

- Step One: Let's discuss the definition:
  - What stands out in the statement?
  - What do you know about the statement?
  - What is happening in the text?
  - What kind of text is this?

- Step Two: What does the Bible say?
  - What is the world like in this passage?
  - What human predicament is revealed?
  - What indicates a change of mind, heart, or behavior?
  - What gives celebration for the world?
  - What does the Bible or church tradition say about health?

- Step Three: What does your own experience say about this?
  - How do you identify with this passage?
  - Can you recall a time in your life where you felt or did not feel this way?
  - What are your thoughts and feelings on this definition?
  - What does your health mean to you in light of our conversation?
  - In what way does your faith support, inform, or challenge you in light of this definition?

- Step Four: What does our culture (the world around us) say about health?

- Step Five: What is your position on health?
  - Where do you stand?
  - "I believe. . . ."
- Step Six: Insights and Implications

Conclusion

Wrap-Up
Leader's Talking Points:

- How's your walking going?
- What goals will you make to become healthier?

Close with Prayer

Week 4: Meditation and Health or Nutrition and Health

Gather

Open with Prayer

Presentation and Discussion

Activity Choice A: Meditation and Health
Leader's Talking Points:
Facilitate a period of meditation or walk a labyrinth for this week's activity. Discuss the group's experience.

Activity Choice B: Nutrition and Health: Meals with Jesus
Leader's Talking Points:
Discuss the joy of food. Discuss that Jesus is always eating and drinking in the Bible. There is prayer at the table. There is laughter, and tears, and talking. They are sitting down and they are devoted to one another. No one is eating meal replacement bars or drinks. They are eating real food and they are thrilled to be at Jesus' table. If you have a health background, discuss what healthy eating means. Eat real food, in moderation and with joy.

- Give each group a poster board or newsprint. Have them discuss as a group a menu they would prepare for Jesus.
- Ask each group to share their meal with the larger group and tell WHY they chose this menu to share with Jesus.
- How would it feel to eat a meal with Jesus? What would it mean to you?
- As a group, names foods or meals that occur in the Bible. What do you think about the different biblical meals and the food that God gives us in the Bible?

Conclusion

Wrap-Up

- Thoughts?
- Questions?

Close with Prayer

Week 5: Where Do We Go From Here?

Gather

Open with Prayer

Presentation and Discussion

Activity: Slipping-Up Discussion
Leader's Talking Points

- Throughout your life, when you gave something up, did you make your goal?
- Have you stuck to your walking challenge? Did you meet your goals?
- How has it felt to walk with Christ?
- Is it hard? Christ's life was hard.
- So what? What do we do when we slip up?

Let's brainstorm some ideas of what we can do when we slip up:

- Get back on the wagon
- Pray
- Ask forgiveness
- Revaluate your goals—are they unattainable? Is it really what Christ is calling you to do?
- Other ways to improve self-discipline
- Stick with your Christ Walk buddies and continue these healthy practices throughout the year, not just during Lent or this study. Encourage each other on each person's journey to healthier life. We each make each other better Christians.

Conclusion

Wrap-Up

- Give thanks to God for the opportunity each day to improve our wellbeing
- Questions?
- Don't forget to keep plugging away with miles!
- Thank you! Good Luck!

Close with Prayer

Week 6: Conclusion/Graduation/Healthy Potluck (optional):

Host a healthy potluck and challenge your participants to bring a healthy dish and recipe to share.

- Give thanks to God for the opportunity each day to improve our wellbeing
- Recap the last five weeks.
- Offer the opportunity to share experiences
- Questions?
- Don't forget to keep plugging away with miles!
- Thank you! Good Luck!
- Awards (optional): You can make up awards, get water bottles with your church logo or t-shirts depending on your budget, and give to the participants. You can also create a satisfaction survey if you would like.

Close with the Christ Walk Prayer (p. 125)

Example 2
Walking with Christ: A Six-Week Program of Theological Reflection

Week 1: Introducing Christ Walk

Week 2: Creation and the Body

Week 3: Sin and the Body

Week 4: Judgment and the Body

Week 5: Repentance and the Body

Week 6: Redemption and the Body

Week 1: Introducing Christ Walk
Gather

Open with Prayer
You can assign weekly prayer duties to each of the teams in your group if you have a large enough group, or ask volunteers to lead opening and closing prayer each week.

Introduce an Ice Breaker

Presentation and Discussion
Leader's Talking Points:

- We are called to walk with Christ in our everyday life
- Mind, body, and spirit
- Each day we should resolve to walk with Christ
- "This is the day that the Lord has made, let us rejoice and be glad in it."
- We can use the Holy Spirit to work towards better mind, body, and spiritual health

We'll be using the actual motion of "walking with Christ" during this challenge and goal towards better mind, body, and spiritual health. This goal will be a metaphor for many changes in our lives and how we are called to serve Christ, how we stick with it, how we might slip up, and how we take this on to the rest of our lives.

With this challenge you begin your commitment to walk with Christ.

- You will choose a walking challenge to work on during Lent (or whatever time frame you have chosen).

- You can choose to pair up with a buddy to work together towards your walk with Christ.

- You will choose an individual goal and your group will choose a group goal. (This is a good time to distribute the Christ Walk books and check out the appendices.)

- There is room in the back of your book to track your daily miles towards your goal.

- Each day in your book includes a journal space to help you on your way:
  - Spaces to record distance
  - Spaces to record reflective thoughts on journey
  - Daily prayers and thoughts on a Christ-centered life

Considerations for Walking

- You may use a pedometer (step counter) to measure your distance each day. Approximately 2,000 to 2,500 steps equals 1 mile. (Option: Distribute pedometers to each participant.)

- You do not have to walk; you can use a treadmill, run, bike, swim, or whatever activity you can measure in terms of miles.

- If you cannot measure mileage, roughly fifteen minutes of physical activity (like an aerobics class) equals one mile. The important thing is to choose something to be physically active.

- Document miles in mile tracker in Christ Walk—there is a table in the back of the book to use *(see page 220)*.

- If you get a pedometer or a Fitbit or other fitness-tracking device (available at places like Target, Wal-Mart or any other sporting goods store), we can discuss use at the next class. Otherwise, start keeping track of the steps and miles you are taking with your new fitness tracker.

Activity: Your Walking Team

- Break into team(s)
- Brainstorm team name
- Develop short team prayer
- Agree on team walking goal
- Share with the larger group

Conclusion

Wrap-Up:

- Review mind, body, and spiritual journey
- Develop a Christ-centered life through mind, body, and spiritual exercises (exercise, study, healthy eating, prayer and/or meditation!)
- Questions?

Homework:

- Choose a walking challenge
- Meditate on the purpose of your goal and the change you want to happen in the next six weeks
- Purchase pedometer, or Fitbit, or other fitness tracker
- Pray for your team

Close with Prayer

Week 2: Creation and the Body

Gather

Open with Prayer

Presentation and Discussion

Leader's Talking Points

- What does society say about creation? How does the secular world define creation?
- What does the church/tradition say about creation? How did God create us?
- What are our conflicts about these two, possibly opposing, views?
- What insights have we had from this discussion?

Use newsprint to capture people's comments/notes. Make a quad chart on the paper:

- In upper right corner write: Society
- In the upper left corner write: Church/Tradition
- In the lower right corner write: What is the conflict between these two beliefs about creation?
- In the lower left corner write: Conclusions/Insights

Facilitate a group discussion of what creation means based on these four different aspects of creation.

Conclusion

Close with Prayer

Week 3: Sin and the Body

Gather

Open with Prayer

Presentation and Discussion

Leader's Talking Points

- What is sin?
- What does sin look like?
- How do we sin in regards to our health?
- What does the Bible say about sin?
- What does society say about sin?
- How does this make us feel?
- Do we feel connected between our physical health and our spiritual health?
- Do we consider our health habits sins?

Method 1: Open a discussion using the questions above and facilitate a conversation using these questions. You can capture thoughts and feelings and consensus from the group on your presentation paper. Close with any insights and comments.

Method 2: Use the Quad Chart method from "Creation." In each corner write:

- What does sin look like?
- What does society say about sin and the body?
- Do we consider our health habits sins?
- How do we feel about this?
- Capture the participants' comments in each quadrant of the chart.
- Close with any final comments and insights.

Conclusion

Close with Prayer

Week 4: Judgment and the Body

Gather

Open with Prayer

Presentation and Discussion

Leader's Talking Points
  What is judgment?

- What are the differences between biblical judgment and social judgment? (You can split newsprint in two columns: One with a heading of "biblical judgment" and the other with "social judgment." Capture the participants' comments. See where the discussion leads and then draw the group around to the next topic.

- Do you feel that poor health is an example of judgment?

- Why or why not? (You can use the column method above and discuss why or why not poor health is an example of judgment.) It is very important to facilitate this carefully and nonjudgmentally, reminding the group that everyone's feelings and thoughts are important. Not everyone will agree about this topic. Discuss it lovingly and kindly and remind the group that no one person is correct.

- How does judgment make you feel about God?

- How do we move away from judgment or accept judgment in our lives?

Conclusion

Leader's Talking Points

- Pray about judgment in your life!
- What comes after judgment? Repentance!
- Pray, walk, record/journal, and move!

Close with Prayer

Week 5: Repentance and the Body

Gather

Open with Prayer

Presentation and Discussion

Leader's Talking Points

You may choose to capture the comments on newsprint. This often helps people gain insights from the discussion.

- Recap what we have discovered about our health so far.
- What does repentance mean to you?
- What does repentance of our health habits mean?
- How is that tied to a godly life? Why should what we do physically matter to our spiritual wellness?
- Does it matter?
- How do we show that we are repentant?
- Do you think God cares what we eat, whether we exercise, or if we have healthy habits?
- It is important to realize that the choices you make today will largely determine how healthy you are tomorrow.

Conclusion

Close with Prayer

Week 6: Redemption and the Body

Gather

Open with Prayer

Presentation and Discussion

Leader's Talking Points

Divide a sheet of newsprint in two columns. In one column write: What is redemption of the body? In another column write: What is redemption of the soul? Compare and contrast. Capture insights and similarities on another piece of paper. Other questions for consideration:

- Do you feel you are redeemed?
- Do you feel you are worthy of redemption?
- Do you feel that your health habits lead to a healthier spiritual life?
- Where do we go from here on this journey?
- How do we share our message of redemption, body, mind, and soul, with others?

Conclusion

Close with Prayer

Bibliography

Bachman, Keith L. "Obesity, Weight Management, and Health Care Costs: A Primer." *Disease Management*. 10:3 (2007): 129–137.

Bowman, Shanthy A. "Television-Viewing Characteristics of Adults: Correlations to Eating Practices and Overweight and Health Status," *Preventing Chronic Disease*, 3:2 (2006), 1–11. Accessed on January 29, 2008 from www.cdc.gov/pcd/issues/2006/apr/05_0139.htm.

Green, Beverly B., Allen Cheadle, Adam S. Pellegrini, and Jeffrey Harris. "Active for Life: A Work Based Physical Activity Program. "*Preventing Chronic Disease*" (2007). Accessed on June 18, 2007 from http://www.cdc.gov/pcd/issues/2007/jul/06_0065.htm.

Isaacs, A.J., J.A. Critchley, S.S.Tai, K. Buckingham, D. Westley, S.D.R. Harridge, C. Smith, and J.M. Gottlieb. "Exercise Evaluation Randomized Trial (EXERT): A Randomized trial comparing GP referral for leisure centre-based exercise, community-based walking and advice only." *Health Technology Assessment*. 11:10 (2007), 1–185.

Jakicic, J.M., and A.D. Otto. "Motivating Change: Modifying Eating and Exercise Behaviors for Weight Management." *American College of Sports Medicine Health and Fitness Journal*, 9:1 (2005), 6–12.

Musich, S., T. McDonald, D. Hirschland, and D. Edington. "Examination of Risk Status Transitions Among Active Employees in a Comprehensive Worksite Health Promotion Program." *Journal of Occupational and Environmental Medicine*. 45:4 (2003), 393–399.

Polascsek M., L.M. O'Brien, W. Lagasse, and N. Hammar. "Move & Improve: a worksite wellness program in Maine." *Prevention of Chronic Disease* (2006). Accessed on June 18, 2007 from http://www.cdc.gov/pcd/issues/2006/jul/05_0123.htm.

Samuelson, M. "Stages of change: From theory to practice." *The Art of Health Promotion* 2: 5 (1998): 1–12.

Steps and Mileage Tracker

You can use the following space to track your progress through your challenge. Each day, add in your steps for the day, the miles for the day, and then add that into the total column for a running total of your progress. You can also make copies of these pages to use in subsequent challenges! Enjoy your journey!

Date	Steps	Miles	Today's Total	Running Total

Date	Steps	Miles	Today's Total	Running Total